Kim Lyons'
Your Body, Your Life

The 12-Week Program
to Optimum Physical,
Mental & Emotional Fitness

KIM LYONS &
LARA McGLASHAN

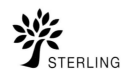

STERLING

New York / London
www.sterlingpublishing.com

STERLING and the distinctive Sterling logo are registered trademarks
of Sterling Publishing Co., Inc.

Library of Congress Cataloging-in-Publication Data Available

10   9   8   7   6   5   4   3   2

Published by Sterling Publishing Co., Inc.
387 Park Avenue South, New York, NY 10016
© 2007 by Kim Lyons and Lara McGlashan
Distributed in Canada by Sterling Publishing
c/o Canadian Manda Group, 165 Dufferin Street
Toronto, Ontario, Canada M6K 3H6
Distributed in the United Kingdom by GMC Distribution Services
Castle Place, 166 High Street, Lewes, East Sussex, England BN7 1XU
Distributed in Australia by Capricorn Link (Australia) Pty. Ltd.
P.O. Box 704, Windsor, NSW 2756, Australia

Book design and layout: *tabula rasa* graphic design
Illustrations: Robin Williams

Printed in China
All rights reserved

Sterling ISBN-13: 978-1-4027-5142-4
          ISBN-10: 1-4027-5142-7

For information about custom editions, special sales, premium and
corporate purchases, please contact Sterling Special Sales
Department at 800-805-5489 or specialsales@sterlingpublishing.com.

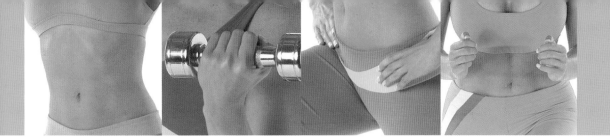

Contents

Foreword by John Kasik | iv

Foreword by Micheal A. Clark | v

Acknowledgments | vi

Prologue | viii

It's All About YOU! | 1

Chapter 1. **YOUR GEAR** | 2

Chapter 2. **YOUR BODY, FROM THE INSIDE OUT** | 5

Chapter 3. **YOUR MIND** | 15

Chapter 4. **YOUR GOALS** | 21

Chapter 5. **YOUR JOURNALS** | 29

Chapter 6. **YOUR FITNESS** | 35

Your Workout! | 45

Chapter 7. **UNDERSTAND IT** | 46

Chapter 8. **PLAN IT** | 52

Chapter 9. **WORK IT** | 59

    Level I Moves | 63

    Level II Moves | 95

    Level III Moves | 127

    Stretching Moves | 159

Chapter 10. **INJURY PREVENTION** | 175

Your Nutrition! | 183

Chapter 11. **THE BAD FAD** | 184

Chapter 12. **BACK TO BASICS** | 190

Chapter 13. **BEYOND THE BASICS** | 196

Chapter 14. **THE DEAL WITH MEALS** | 206

Chapter 15. **GROCERY SHOPPING
AND MEAL PLANNING** | 214

Chapter 16. **KIM'S RECIPES** | 222

Your Future! | 241

Chapter 17. **REASSESS AND REEVALUATE** | 242

Chapter 18. **GLITCHES AND GAINS** | 248

Chapter 19. **MAINTAINING MOTIVATION** | 256

Epilogue | 260

Index | 261

Foreword
by John Kasik

Americans are obsessed with weight. All it takes is a stroll through the supermarket checkout to deduce just how much this obsession impacts our daily lives. Every magazine in the rack touts a new weight-loss trend or magical celebrity diet, or lays out scandalous news and photographs about which movie stars are too fat or too thin. While this obsession certainly isn't healthy, it has made shows like *The Biggest Loser* successful. But to me, this is a boon rather than a drawback, because unlike much reality television out there, *The Biggest Loser* promotes something real and life altering—an opportunity to lose weight once and for all through sensible diet and exercise routines.

In 2006, Kim Lyons was introduced to this program and to me, as I was the on-site athletic trainer for the contestants at the time. I watched along with millions of viewers as Kim encouraged, cajoled, and inspired her team to lose incredible amounts of weight, literally changing the course of their lives in only a few short months. Every week, we watched in awe as the Red Team struggled through transformations not only of body but also of mind and spirit, and Kim was there, supporting and encouraging them through a roller coaster of emotions and physical changes. Now, I've worked as a certified athletic trainer for professional athletes for more than twenty years, and even though it was their job to be athletes, it was hard even for them to be dedicated and committed to

such a program! I can only imagine how difficult it was for those on *The Biggest Loser* ranch. But they had what many people don't—a personal trainer who cared about them and helped them through one of the hardest periods in their lives: Kim Lyons. Now you, too, can have the same advantage the Red Team has season after season—the benefit of Kim's wisdom and experience at your fingertips.

In *Your Body, Your Life*, Kim leads you by the hand through the process of weight loss, much in the same way she does her television contestants, offering solid information, encouraging advice, and fun stories to help you push through and persevere. Kim is as committed to helping you change your life as she is to helping her Red Team contestants change theirs, and will help you accomplish your goals one calorie at a time, one rep at a time. Just like it works for those on television, so can it work for you, too.

So open this book and lose weight the "Red Team" way. Take advantage of this opportunity and change the direction of your life for the better!

John Kasik, MS, ATC, Cped,
Head Athletic Trainer,
Stanford University

Foreword
by Micheal A. Clark

Kim's relationship with the National Academy of Sports Medicine (NASM) began more than ten years ago when she completed her personal training certification. At NASM we focus on an evidence-based approach to fitness, built on a foundation of comprehensive scientific research supported by leading institutes and universities. By completing our certification, Kim Lyons proved she had a solid grasp of programming, technique, and motivation when it comes to personal fitness.

For more than a decade, Kim has excelled in the world of fitness. She has been physically active her whole life and has inspired, motivated, and uplifted countless clients through the years. As a trainer on NBC's *The Biggest Loser,* Kim uses her positive attitude, solid training methodology, and comprehensive nutritional tips to garner her contestants fantastic results!

Because of her various experiences, Kim has a unique perspective on fitness. She realizes the time constraints we all face and knows how difficult it is to fit an effective workout regime into our busy schedules. Her book, *Your Body, Your Life,* now makes it possible to live a fit lifestyle! By following her simple strategies, anyone of any size can work out and be well on their way to weight loss and overall healthier living. Her easy-to-understand approach focuses on circuit training, of which I have long been an advocate. Circuit training is an excellent strategy for

developing good basic strength and body tone, delivering effective results in a short amount of time. Kim's circuit workouts will elevate your heart rate, develop muscle tone, and enable you to get your workouts done quickly and efficiently.

As a doctor of physical therapy and president and CEO of NASM, I see clients struggle every day to maintain their weight, improve muscle strength, and build endurance. I'm confident that Kim's recommendations on diet and exercise will allow individuals, regardless of age or fitness level, to accomplish their goals. I recommend her book to anyone who wants to make lasting changes to their bodies and their lives. No matter what your abilities, let Kim Lyons be your motivational fitness coach, and you'll undoubtedly achieve sustainable, healthy results. As the title of the book conveys, it's *Your Body, Your Life*!

Yours in health,
Micheal A. Clark, DPT, MS, PES, CES
President and CEO, NASM

Acknowledgments

Someone once told me that life resembles a football game. The quarterback throws the winning touchdown, but without the rest of his team working hard to make that winning play happen, he could never be a hero. In much the same way, I could never have written this book without the love, support, encouragement, and inspiration from those on my own team, and they deserve to share the glory of this touchdown with me.

To Mom and Dad: Thank you for always making me eat my broccoli and kicking me outside to play when I wanted to watch TV! Your support and love has made a difference in my life, a difference I will try to pass on to millions of people.

To my grandma: You've always given me support, believed in my craziest dreams, and helped me find beauty in every sunset, even on rainy days. You truly are an inspiration to the world.

To my big sister, Debby: Thank you tons for your years of patience and understanding, and for helping me be less of a goofball in the world. You've always given me love when I probably deserved a swift kick in the butt!

To my superhero husband: You helped me let go of the safety bar on the roller coaster of life. Together we can do anything! We've only begun, baby . . . hold on tight!

To NBC, Reveille, and 3-Ball: Thank you for seeing potential in me I never knew I possessed! I am only one of the millions of lives you have touched through *The Biggest Loser* and am so proud to be part of this journey.

To all of my clients and "Red Team Peeps": Your strength and dedication inspires me to do what I do. We have sweat, cried, laughed, and brawled together, and I'll never forget our experiences.

To my Sterling family for making my vision a reality: Thank you, Jo and Charlie, for your dedication and expertise in making my first book everything I dreamed it would be and more!

To Julie and Courtney: Thanks for helping me explore the possibilities I never knew existed and becoming part of my wonderful team!

To my literary agent, Joy: For guiding my little "gym rat" self through the streets of New York and making this process so fun and understandable!

To NASM and my Weider family: For your knowledge, research, and support. You've given me the gift to help change lives.

To Donna, Krystal, and Cory: Special thanks for helping me look pretty, stylish, and not 10 pounds heavier on film! Cheers to (almost) no diva moments!

To Elisabetta Rogiani: Thanks for the fabulous workout and cover outfits! They were exactly what I envisioned.

And last, but by far not least, to my best friend and co-author, Lara: You've done it! You have taken ten years of my crazy thoughts and ideas and made them come together on paper. We have come a long way from our days of running the Galaxy Obstacle Course together! You have relentlessly pushed me to be my best, and I am forever grateful for your support and endless belief in me. Without you, this book would remain just another idea! You are the only one who can finish my sentences and dot my i's while I cross the t's. (Wait, did I do that yet? I can't remember. Can you check?) I can't wait to see what adventures the next ten years bring!

For more information on those who helped put this book together, please visit these Web sites:

Writing:
Lara McGlashan
www.laramcglashan.com

Photography:
Cory Sorensen
www.corysorensen.com

Styling:
Krystal Debord
www.krystaldebord.com

Wardrobe:
Elisabetta Rogiani
www.rogiani.com

Hair and makeup:
Donna Gast
www.donnagast.com

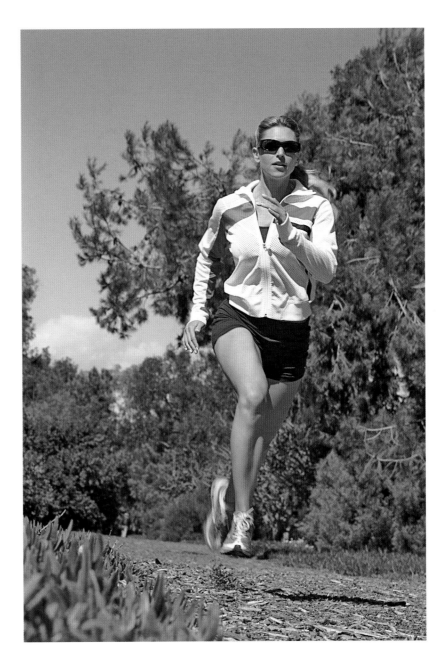

Prologue

Dear Readers,

Welcome to *Your Body, Your Life*! I am so excited to have this opportunity to share the gift of health and fitness with you! Through my time-tested, fat-burning circuit training system and my solid, comprehensive nutrition program, you'll learn how to lose weight once and for all, breaking free of that destructive yo-yo dieting pattern that messes with your head, your metabolism, and your body image.

Your Body, Your Life breaks down all the aspects of fitness and weight loss in an uncomplicated and understandable way. Using this book as your guide, you'll start exercising, eating correctly, and losing weight right away! In addition, you'll come to understand the emotional side of weight loss and will learn how your body and your mind are intimately connected. Many of my clients (some from television, some not) have been good enough to share their emotional experiences with me for this book. Their stories are touching, funny, and uplifting, and I am sure you'll find hope and inspiration in their tales.

At the end of each chapter you'll find a section called Homework. Each homework item helps you achieve a goal of some kind, be it mental, physical, or emotional, reinforcing a lot of the key points you'll be learning as you read through the book. I highly encourage you to do the homework, not only because you'll learn a ton about your body and your mind, but also because you'll feel a sense of accomplishment each time you complete an item!

While it would be great if you read *Your Body, Your Life* from cover to cover, I expect you'll want to flip around, skip ahead, and read things you may be particularly interested in at the moment. That's cool with me! But make sure you eventually read everything in here, because you may just learn something about yourself you didn't expect. I want you to use this book not only as a starting point for a lifetime of fitness but also as a reference that you can turn to time and again for inspiration, ideas, and motivation.

Enough chitchat—let's get started!

Love,
Kim

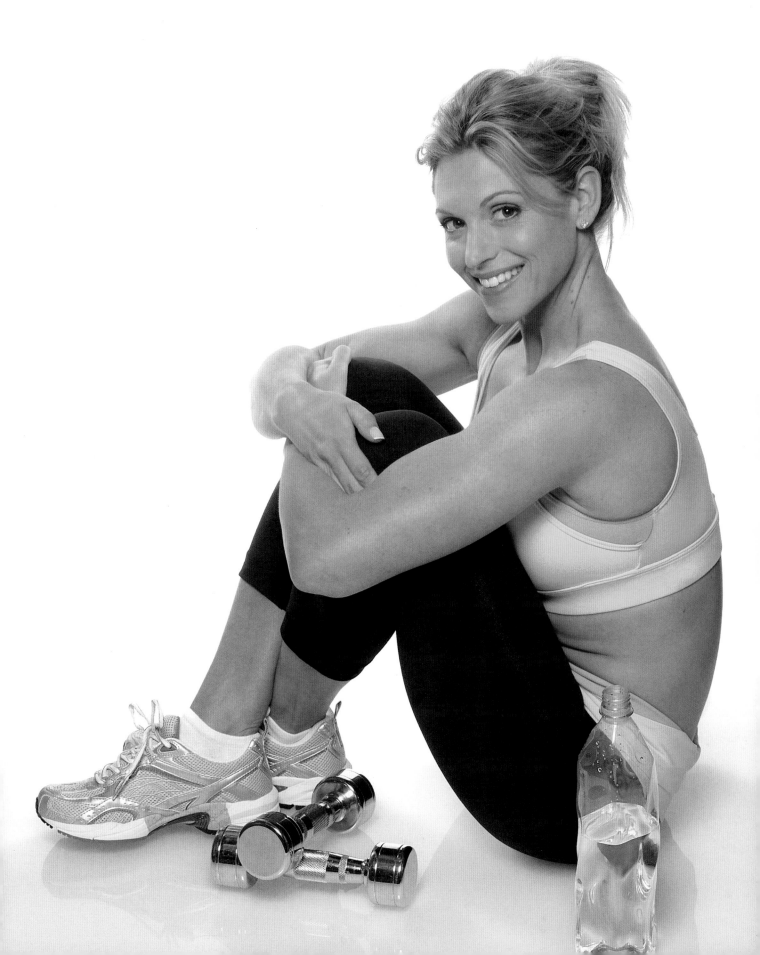

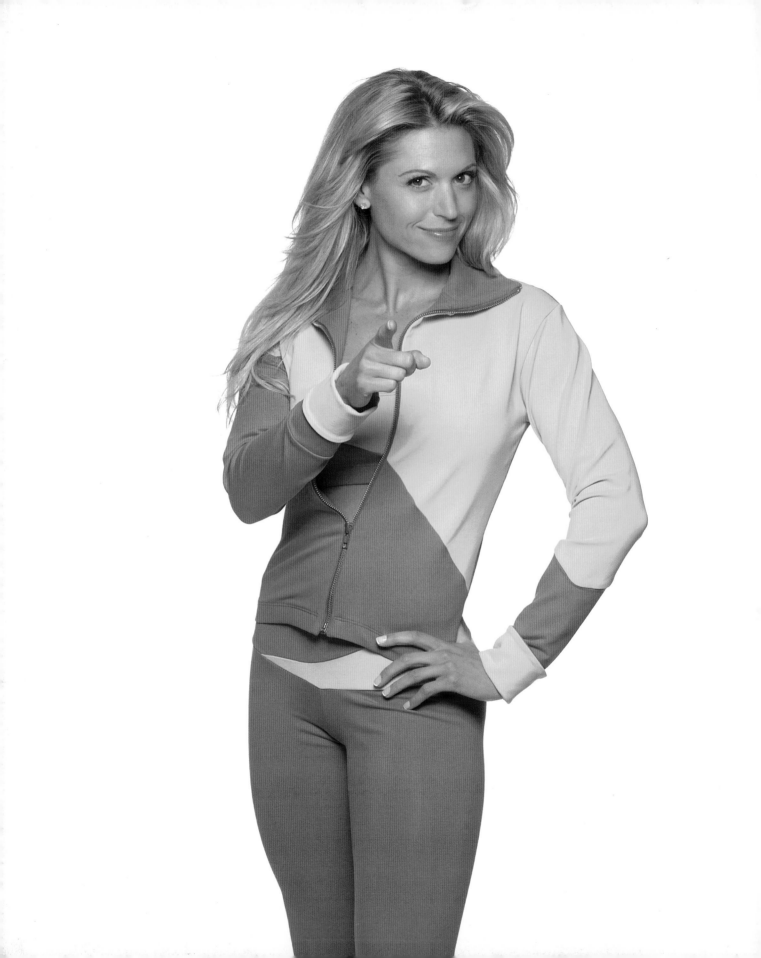

It's All About YOU!

WELCOME TO YOUR NEW LIFE! This may sound hokey, but making the decision to start a fitness program is like a rebirth. You're literally giving up your old self and replacing it with a new one! In the next twelve weeks, you'll shed your old ways of eating and living and replace them with new, healthy habits and emotions. You'll also be giving up your negative ideas about yourself and your body and trading them for positive, uplifting thoughts. This new, fit life offers so many exciting possibilities, it's hard not to be stoked!

This section is all about *you* and will help you get to know intimately the body you'll be changing. In these pages you'll come to understand the inner workings of your mind and body and will get mentally and physically ready to start your new, fit lifestyle!

CHAPTER 1

Your Gear

A lot of you probably want to start working out right now! If so, turn to Chapter 9, page 59, read the instructions, and do Level I, Circuit 1 right now, with or without weights! For those of you in less of an extreme hurry, here's what you'll need in the coming weeks:

DUMBBELLS

You're going to need a few sets of dumbbells of varying weights because as you get stronger you'll need heavier resistance. I recommend starting with 2- or 3-pound dumbbells and working your way up to 5-, 8-, or even 10-pound weights over the course of twelve weeks.

ATHLETIC SHOES

Good news, girls—you get to go shoe shopping! I recommend buying a solid pair of cross trainers for the *Your Body, Your Life* workout program. Cross trainers can be used for a variety of different activities and offer good all-around support. Not everyone fits in all brands, depending on the shape of your feet. For example, New Balance shoes generally have a wide toe box and are good for people with wide feet, whereas Puma shoes are typically narrower. Try on several brands in the store and walk around in them for 5 minutes to see whether they're comfortable and fit correctly.

BURNING QUESTION

Is there really a difference between a fifty-dollar and a hundred-dollar pair of sneakers?
Sometimes. If the shoe is trendy or popular among teenagers, its price is probably driven by fashion rather than functionality. But sometimes, the higher sticker price is based on new shoe technology. I have to admit, I am a cheapo when it comes to buying athletic shoes, but sometimes they're worth the extra expense. I bought a stupidly expensive pair of Nikes for *The Biggest Loser*, season 3 (mostly because they were red!). But they were incredible! So good, in fact, I had the network buy all

my contestants the same shoes. This is not to say that you should go out and buy a horribly expensive pair of shoes because I said to. (I still think that sticker price was way too high for a pair of running shoes!) But remember that your body, joints, and feet are going to be impacted by these shoes for the next twelve weeks, so get the best, most solid shoe you can comfortably afford.

WATER BOTTLE

Whether you're using a plain plastic Evian bottle or a pop-top rubber bicycle bottle, this bad boy is your new best friend. For the next twelve weeks, you'll be taking water with you everywhere—to work, in your car, to the gym, everywhere. You'll get so you feel lost without it!

MIRROR

I recommend buying a cheap, full-length mirror and hanging it in the room you're going to be using for your workouts. This mirror is a great tool, especially if you're just learning how to exercise. Using the mirror, you'll easily be able to check your exercise form and correct any errors you're making.

CLOTHING

Wear comfortable, supportive clothing that is not restrictive, but also that is not too baggy. Baggy clothes have a tendency

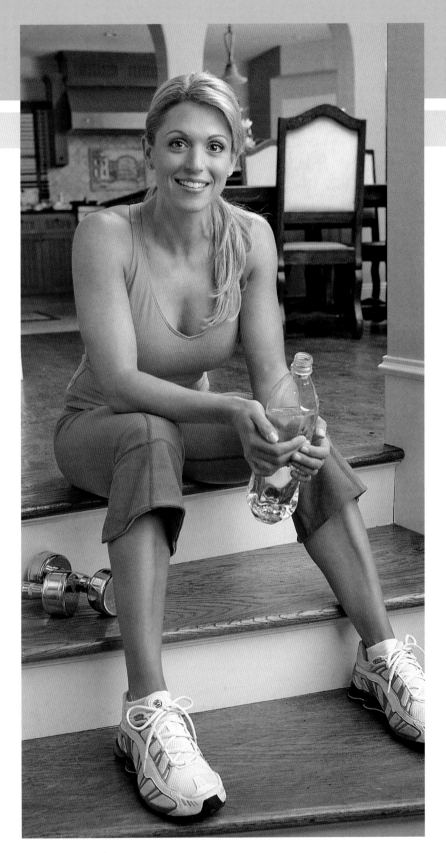

to bunch up and rub in sensitive areas. Many of my clients have trouble with chafing, especially between their legs. Simple biker or Lycra shorts are a favorite for solving this problem, as they allow the legs to slide by each other without much friction. A good sports bra is a must, as are good socks. Buy clothing and socks that contain a blend of synthetic fibers to pull sweat away from the body and the feet to help prevent blisters, chafing, and athlete's foot.

BURNING QUESTION

How do I find a good sports bra? This is the million-dollar question! Sports bras are an essential piece of clothing, especially if you're well-endowed up top. They'll hold your breasts in place while you exercise, preventing pain and damage to the supporting tissue. Most bras are "compression"-type garments, meaning they hold your breasts down with a tight band of elastic fabric. Some, however, offer supportive cups as well as compression for more full-busted women. Although there are plenty of them out there, it takes a lot of trial and error to find a sports bra that fits you correctly and comfortably. Try on a number of different bras and see what feels good. Jump up and down in the store and see how the bra holds up—literally! A good bra should be supportive without being restrictive and should never pinch or be painful. Personally, I love Champion brand sports bras because they fit me in all the right places.

TOWEL

A must for those of you who tend to "glow" heavily when working out. A small hand towel will do the trick nicely.

JOURNALS

You're going to need two separate journals for the *Your Body, Your Life* program, one for your workouts and one for your food. These can be any sort of paper product you like, from a fifty-cent spiral notepad to a pricier manufactured journal bought from the bookstore. A lot of my clients like to buy purse-size journals they can pop in their handbag and carry with them. And a note for people who aren't big on writing things down: Do it anyhow! Your entries don't have to be essays or insightful commentaries on life's foibles! They can be simple notes jotted down quickly at the end of the day that record how you did, how you felt, and so forth. You'll be really glad to have those journals later on; trust me.

SUMMARY

Simply getting "geared up" can help motivate you to start your new lifestyle. Stock up on all your new equipment and clothing as soon as possible, and you'll be ready to roll mentally and physically!

HOMEWORK

1. Go shopping! Buy new clothing and shoes for your workouts, snap up a few sets of dumbbells, and buy a couple of journals for good measure.
2. Clear out a workout space in your home for your new gear! This will be the space you'll be using to work out for the next twelve weeks, so make sure you've got plenty of room to move around.
3. Today and the rest of this week, take a small walk around the neighborhood. Nothing big—just 10–15 minutes of strolling around to get your body moving! To learn more about the importance of cardio activity, turn to page 49.

CHAPTER 2

Your Body, from the Inside Out

Most of you are probably unhappy with your body. Whether you think you're too fat, too short, too bottom heavy, or too busty, you probably purchased this book hoping to change your body for the better. I think this is great! You're being proactive and doing something to incite change instead of being passive, resigning yourself to misery.

This chapter is dedicated to helping you understand the inner workings of your body, which in turn will help you formulate concrete goals and develop realistic expectations about your ultimate results. While reading this chapter, try to step back and look at your body objectively and without prejudice. It's so easy to get caught up in hating your body and how it looks that you can easily forget how incredible it really is, but if you think about it, it can blow your mind! I mean, just while I am sitting here writing,

my body is digesting breakfast, thinking about words, moving my fingers, breathing, pumping blood, creating hormones— and a myriad of other incredible feats, all on its own! Yet as incredible as it is, you may still find it difficult to appreciate your body, when all you see in the mirror is a source of unhappiness and pain. But for better or for worse, this is your only body, the vessel you've been given to take you through life. It's up to you to nurture it, cherish it, and make it the best body possible.

Open your mind to the possibility that your body is incredible and capable of amazing things. This might be hard to do, especially if you're used to putting yourself down or entertaining negative thoughts about yourself. But know this: There is nothing wrong or horrible about who you are. You and your body are unique and amazing! Once you understand how your body works, looks, and responds, you'll be better able to achieve the goals you'll be making and can finally have the body you've always wanted. Okay? Let's get to it!

YOUR GENETICS

Clients often come to me and say, "I want legs like Cindy Crawford's, a booty like J-Lo's, and abs like Fergie's!" And I say, "Sheesh, me, too!" But a word to the wise: It's not gonna happen. In the real world, genetics reign supreme.

Your genetics dictate everything about you—your hair color, your eye color, your height, your shape, and to a certain extent your weight. But ultimately, your eating and exercise habits determine your weight; your genetics simply determine where that weight is stored. Some bodies like to put extra fat around the waist, others around the butt and thighs. These genetic fat "depositories" tend to become a source of obsession, and there isn't a woman out there who doesn't have her own "trouble spots" she would love to eliminate. But genetics aren't all bad, and we've all got good qualities we can flaunt and be proud of. You've just got to work with what God—and your parents—have given you, recognizing and appreciating your good traits instead of obsessing over what you consider your less attractive ones. Accept who you are, then work with what you've got to create the best you possible.

BURNING QUESTION

My whole family is overweight. Does this mean I am genetically doomed to be overweight, too? Absolutely not. Genetics have very little to do with how fat you are, and anyone who says differently will say so while eating a handful of chips. Families tend to be overweight together because they eat the same bad foods and live the same sedentary lifestyle. Your genetics can't control what you eat or how much you exercise, so don't use them as a crutch for being excessively overweight. Because no matter where your body likes to store its extra fat— hips, thighs, or waist—you're the one putting that cupcake in your mouth, giving it more fat to store! Many times, I have seen entire overweight families turn themselves around and become as fit together as they were fat together, proving that their problem was lifestyle induced rather than genetic.

YOUR BODY TYPE

Your genetics also dictate your body shape—whether you've got long arms or short legs, a high waist or big breasts. A lot of people run into trouble when they model their physique and weight-loss goals after someone with a completely different body type than their own. For example, I love Jennifer Garner's body—love her legs, love her arms, love everything! But if I try to model my own body after hers, I will constantly be disappointed. I look nothing like her either in skeletal frame or body composition, and no matter how hard I try, I will never have legs like hers. Of course, I can make improvements to my own legs, but I have to be real about what my legs will look like when they are at their most fit, because even then, they will still not look like Jennifer Garner's legs.

So let's get real: What do you look like? What do your genetics dictate in terms of body type? Generally speaking, people fall into three different body types: ectomorph, endomorph, and mesomorph. Look at each of these types carefully and see which of them best matches your own body. Recognizing your body type will give you realistic parameters with which

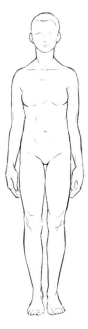

Ectomorph

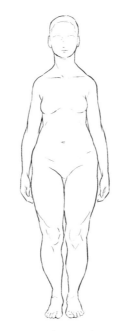

Endomorph

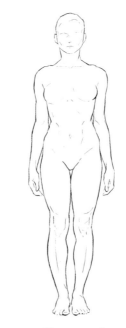

Mesomorph

to work when deciding on exercise and weight-loss goals as well as appropriate physical role models.

Ectomorph

Ectomorphs are long, lean, and lanky, with small bones, narrow hips, and a small waist. They usually have a hard time gaining weight, especially muscle, and lack feminine curves. This "boy body" type is the one most fashion models have, and their legs are usually longer than their torsos.

Endomorph (apple shaped)

Endomorphs have heavier bones and thicker waists and accumulate fat mainly around their abdomens. Their legs are generally shorter than their torsos, they have more fat than muscle, and they tend to gain weight easily.

Mesomorph (pear shaped)

Mesomorphs fall between the two above extremes. They tend to be athletic and have broad shoulders and hips, narrow waists, and a high percentage of muscle in comparison to fat. Mesomorphs tend to accumulate fat in their lower bodies.

You may not fit perfectly into one of these categories, but see which one best describes your body type, then go with it. Base your workout and diet goals on how your personal body type will look at its most fit instead of trying to force it to become something it's not. But remember: While your genetics may dictate where you store fat, with diet and exercise people of all body types can control how much fat is deposited on their frames!

BURNING QUESTION

How can I do hundreds of sit-ups every day and still have a tummy? Doing hundreds of sit-ups will help you develop a strong core but will do nothing to "spot-reduce" the fat on your tummy. Your body genetically likes to store fat around your abdomen, and while it

Fun Fact

Hate your thunder thighs? Think again. Research has shown that women who carry more fat around their abdomen are at higher risk for heart disease, diabetes, and high blood pressure. So if you're gonna haul around a few extra pounds, it's better to make some thunder down under!

seems logical that you could rid yourself of belly fat by working that place harder than the others, your body does not work that way. When you lose weight, your body draws on fat stores from all over at an even rate. Unfortunately, the places you genetically store the most fat will likely be the last places you lose it. To help reduce your overall body fat, follow a dedicated program of exercise and maintain a healthy diet. And of course, keep up your dedicated ab training! After so many sit-ups, you'll eventually uncover a washboard stomach worthy of turning heads!

BRIGHT IDEA

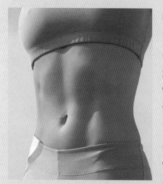

MAKE A COMPLIMENT JOURNAL

For years, I had a very hard time accepting my body type and my genetics for what they were. I always wanted to be model thin, and I referred to my athletic body as "thick" or "chunky." One day I went out to do errands wearing a denim miniskirt, and was mentally berating myself for having chunky, muscular legs, when a woman came up to me and said, "You have the most awesome legs! How do you train them?" That made me feel really good, and I decided to start myself a compliment journal. In it I wrote down nice things people said about me or my body, so on days when I was feeling poorly about myself I could open it up and turn my frown upside down! I recommend this exercise to all my clients who have a poor body image or low self-esteem, because hearing a compliment is one thing, but listening to it and believing it is another animal completely. To help you believe the compliments people give you, it's useful to write them down. Write it down whenever someone tells you how good you look, how smart or funny you are, how great your kids are, or how beautiful your house looks. Whenever you're feeling blue, open your compliment book, read it carefully, and remind yourself how great you really are. A little goes a long way in making you feel good about yourself!

YOUR POSTURE

Your skeletal structure is determined by genetics, and your bones are aligned to stand in a certain way to be strong, stable, and balanced. In exercise terms, this ideal body position is called neutral posture.

In this position, all your muscles are contracting in all the right places and your skeleton is fully supported from all angles. This is the posture you want to maintain at work, at home, and while out and about. During exercise, proper posture and correct spinal alignment help absorb shock, prevent fatigue, and place less stress on the joints.

While your skeletal structure is determined by genetics, you are the master of your posture. Some people stand with their hip cocked, or position themselves to hide or flaunt certain body parts, throwing their posture out of whack; other people slouch or stoop all day at work. If your posture constantly deviates from neutral, you'll probably develop muscle weakness, muscle tightness, or a combination of both. These imbalances can cause back, neck, knee, and hip problems if left untreated.

It's important to practice good posture, and I say "practice" because maintaining proper posture can be hard work, especially if you're not used to it. In fact, I have had clients get sore from trying to hold proper posture for long periods of time! No joke. But not only can good posture help you look more confident and outgoing; it also helps prevent muscle imbalances and skeletal weakness.

Stand sideways in front of a mirror and check yourself out. How do you look? Compare yours to some of the common imbalanced postures illustrated on page 9.

Note: These illustrations are extreme examples of deviant postures. You may not notice such a drastic variation in your own stance.

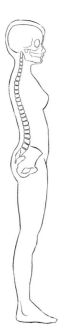

Neutral posture

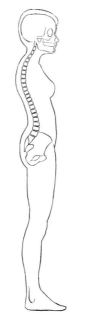

Lordosis posture

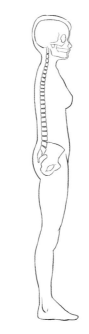

Flat-back posture

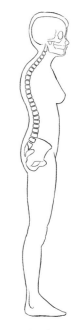

Swayback posture

Lordosis Posture

- **What it looks like:** Your lower back curves inward excessively just above your buttocks, your belly bulges forward, and your butt sticks up higher than normal in the air. Often your shoulders sag and your head juts forward slightly to compensate for the excessive curve in your back.
- **Possible tight muscles:** Hip flexors, lower back
- **Possible weak muscles:** Abs, obliques, glutes, hamstrings

Flat-Back Posture

- **What it looks like:** Your lower back is flat instead of being rounded slightly inward, as is normal. Your butt looks like it's tucked underneath you, and you appear stooped.
- **Possible tight muscles:** Upper abs, glutes, hamstrings
- **Possible weak muscles:** Lower back, hip flexors

Swayback Posture

- **What it looks like:** An excessive arching of the lower back and a roundness (kyphosis) of the upper back. Your hips shoot forward and your torso appears slouched, shoulders rounded forward, and chest sunken in.
- **Possible tight muscles:** Upper abs, hip flexors, pectoral muscles, latissimus dorsi (back muscles)
- **Possible weak muscles:** Obliques, glutes, hamstrings, upper back (rhomboids, trapezius)

Did you find an accurate description of your current posture? If so, then note which muscles you need to work on and keep that in the back of your mind. And remember: no judgment and no worries! No matter what your current posture, you can correct any and all imbalances with dedicated exercise and flexibility training.

Fun Fact
Your BMR accounts for 75–80 percent of your daily energy expenditure!

Want to Know Your Personal BMR?
Go to my website, www.kimlyons.com, and click on "BMR calculator."

BURNING QUESTION

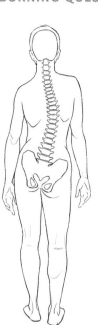

What is scoliosis?

Scoliosis is an abnormal curve of the spine; when viewed from the front, the spine curves to the side. Although the cause of scoliosis is generally unknown, it is believed to be genetic, and most people with scoliosis have been diagnosed by the time they are teenagers. You cannot contract scoliosis—either you have it or you don't. If you suspect you might have it, see your physician before beginning your workout program. He or she may have specific instructions for you to follow with regard to exercise.

Symptoms of Scoliosis

- Your head is off center.
- One hip is higher than the other.
- You might walk with a rolling gait.
- Opposite sides of your body might not seem level.
- You may tire easily when doing abdominal and core movements.

YOUR METABOLISM

Scientifically speaking, your metabolism is a series of chemical reactions in your body that convert the food you eat to energy. Everything you do—breathing, digesting, thinking, even sitting on the couch clicking the remote—requires energy. Your basal metabolic rate (BMR) represents the number of calories (energy) needed to run your body while at rest. Your BMR is influenced by a number of factors: age, height, and gender, which you can't control, and exercise and nutrition, which you can control.

To an extent, your genetics determine your metabolism. Some people are genetically gifted with a high BMR ("fast" metabolism) and can seemingly eat anything and everything and not gain weight. For others, their BMR is either genetically lower ("slow" metabolism) or has been slowed due to age, weight gain, or inactivity. But whether you've got a fast or a slow metabolism, if you're eating more calories than your body needs to run the BMR without offsetting those extra calories with exercise and activity, you're going to gain fat weight. The more weight you gain, the more sedentary you will become and the slower your metabolic rate will get. It's a vicious circle!

The good news is that you can give your metabolism and your BMR a swift kick in the pants! With consistent exercise and healthful eating, you can change your body composition and essentially "reset" your BMR to a higher level. Through resistance training you'll gain lean mass, enabling you to burn more calories at rest, increasing your metabolism. Through consistent exercise, your body will be in a constant cycle of tissue breakdown and repair, requiring energy, again increasing your metabolism and your BMR.

YOUR BODY COMPOSITION

Your body composition is the percentage of fat mass versus the percentage of lean mass you carry around on your frame, and the ultimate goal of any fitness plan is to increase your lean mass while shrinking your fat mass. Some internal body fat, called "essential fat," is necessary for the protection and cushioning of your organs, but the subcutaneous fat stored around your hips, thighs, waist, and abdomen—the stuff we all complain about—is simply excess. When you eat, your body uses the calories it needs right away and puts any extra calories into storage as glycogen or as body fat. To lose excess body fat, you've got to expend more calories than you take in with regular exercise, encouraging the body to use that stored fat as fuel, melting it away.

Your lean mass includes your muscles, bones, and organs. The mass of your organs and bones remains pretty constant, but you can change the size and density of your muscle tissue by working out with weights. The more lean mass you have, the more energy you will burn, even at rest (hence an increase in your BMR!).

Your lifestyle, diet, and exercise habits ultimately determine your body composition. If you're sedentary and eat poorly, you're going to have a high fat mass versus lean mass. If you exercise regularly and eat healthfully, you're going to have more lean mass than fat mass. So what are you waiting for? Put this book down and go for a walk!

BURNING QUESTION

How do I determine my body fat percentage?
The most accurate (and expensive) way is hydrostatic weighing. Here, you are completely submerged in a tank of water and your body density is measured through water displacement. Another way is with skin-fold testing. The tester, usually a gym professional, pinches your skin in several locations and measures these skin folds with calipers, averaging the numbers to determine your body fat percentage. A third way is through bioelectrical impedance analysis (BIA). This is the method used by those "fat-testing" bathroom scales you see for sale everywhere. These scales send a mild electrical current through your body,

Body Fat Percentage Categories

	Women	Men
Essential (internal) fat	10%–12%	2%–4%
Elite athletes	12%–14%	6%–13%
Normal/Acceptable	25%–31%	18%–25%
Obese	32%+	26%+

measuring the "impedance," or resistance to the flow of the current. The more fat you've got, the harder it is for the current to pass through you quickly. The results of the BIA and skin-fold tests can be affected by things such as water retention and human error, so take them with a grain of salt. The results can be as much as 8 percent above or below your actual body fat percentage! Instead of being married to the resultant number, instead focus on lowering that number each week or month. That way, you'll know your body fat is decreasing, even if you're not exactly sure what it is!

Tongue Twister
Instead of saying "I want to get thin," say, "I want to get lean!"

YOUR HEALTH

Many heath problems are genetic—breast cancer, sickle-cell anemia, and type 1 diabetes—but others are self-inflicted. The four most prevalent self-inflicted diseases in America are heart disease, hypertension, obesity, and type 2 diabetes. If you've been inactive and have been making poor food choices for a long period of time, chances are you're at risk for one of these Big Four. Here is what each of the Big Four entails. Believe me, if you weren't committed to your fitness program before, you will be by the end of this section!

- Heart disease is in fact the number one killer of American women!

- More than 300,000 American deaths are linked to obesity every year.

- Hypertension currently affects more than 65 million people—that's 1 in 3 American adults!

- More than 6 million people in the United States have diabetes—*and don't know it*!

A LITTLE MATH

WAIST-TO-HIP RATIO

Use this ratio to determine your fat distribution and overall health risk. People with extra weight around their waist are at greater risk for heart disease and diabetes than those with extra weight around their hips.

1. Measure your waist in line with your belly button.
2. Measure your hips at their widest point.
3. Divide the waist measurement by the hip measurement to get your ratio.

Example: Harriet

Waist: 39

Hip: 33

Ratio = 1.18

The ideal ratio for women is 0.80 (for men it's 0.95). If you're above these ideals, don't worry. As you work out, you'll shrink your accumulated fat stores and will soon be on your way to improving your ratio!

Heart Disease

The bad news: "Heart disease" is a catch-all term describing any disorder of the heart, including angina, coronary artery disease, heart attack, arrhythmia, valve prolapse, and heart failure. Risk factors such as smoking, alcohol consumption, sedentary lifestyle, stress, obesity, hypertension, poor dietary habits, and high cholesterol all contribute to a high risk of heart disease.

The good news: You can significantly reduce your risk of heart disease by changing your lifestyle. Stop smoking, limit alcohol intake, lose weight, eat healthfully, and exercise regularly!

Heart Disease Risk Factors

- age
- gender
- smoking
- hypertension
- diabetes
- artery disease
- high cholesterol
- poor diet
- obesity
- sedentary lifestyle
- alcohol
- drugs

Obesity

The bad news: America is fat. So fat, it's scary. According to the Centers for Disease Control, more than 60 million people in the United States are obese, including 10 million children under the age of eighteen! Obese people are at a higher risk for hypertension, diabetes, heart attack, stroke, and even cancer. Additionally, obesity can lead to gallstones, osteoarthritis, and in some cases, infertility in women.

The good news: In 99.9 percent of cases, obesity is not a permanent condition; it's a voluntary one. As I have proven with my private clients as well as on television, obesity can be successfully reversed with committed exercise and proper nutrition.

Symptoms of Obesity

- a body fat percentage of 32 or higher
- excessive snoring
- recurring heartburn
- aching joints
- depression
- negative self-image

Hypertension (aka High Blood Pressure)

The bad news: Hypertension is a chronic condition in which the pressure put on your vessels by the beating of your heart is constantly elevated, putting you at higher risk for stroke, heart attack, or kidney failure. Hypertension can be caused by high salt intake, obesity, stress, smoking, and excessive alcohol consumption.

The good news: Through diet and lifestyle modification and regular exercise, hypertension can be controlled and even eliminated.

Type 2 Diabetes

The bad news: Because of poor dietary habits and a sedentary lifestyle, type 2 diabetics develop insulin resistance, meaning that insulin cannot get inside their cells to produce energy. As a result, blood sugar increases; if left untreated, this excess blood sugar can damage nerves and blood vessels, which can lead to heart disease, stroke, blindness, kidney disease, and amputation.

The good news: While some of my clients have to take medication for their diabetes, many have reversed their condition with careful diet regulation and regular exercise routines.

Symptoms of Type 2 Diabetes
• increased thirst
• increased hunger
• increased urination
• fatigue
• blurred vision
• sores that don't heal

BURNING QUESTION

What is the difference between type 1 and type 2 diabetes? Both types of diabetes are caused by a problem with insulin, the hormone needed to move glucose (blood sugar) into cells, where it is used for energy. If glucose does not get into the cells, it

remains in the blood, causing the symptoms of diabetes. In type 1 diabetes, the pancreas no longer makes insulin because the body's immune system has attacked and destroyed the cells that create it. These diabetics are usually diagnosed as children or young adults and must take insulin (as injections or a pump) to help control their blood sugar. Many type 1 diabetics can significantly reduce their dependence on medication and improve their condition by making good food choices, exercising regularly, and controlling blood pressure and cholesterol. Type 2 diabetes usually begins with insulin resistance, where cells don't use insulin properly. Soon, the pancreas loses the ability to secrete insulin in response to meals, and glucose accumulates in the blood. Type 2 diabetes can occur at any age, and obese, sedentary people are most likely to develop the disease. Fortunately, many people can reverse or significantly improve their condition with a lifestyle change.

YOUR RESPONSIBILITY

Your body is your responsibility. It's up to you to take care of it to the best of your abilities. This is why everybody—and I mean *everybody*—should go to the doctor regularly and should get a physical once a year. Because sometimes, there can be something seriously wrong with you, even if you don't feel sick. When I first started working on *The Biggest Loser*, I was shocked at how unhealthy my contestants were. Their obesity was obvious, but their internal problems were not. Most of them had high blood pressure and high cholesterol, and some even had early signs of diabetes. And the scariest part: None of them knew they were so sick! They were as shocked as I was when their tests came back from the clinic. Luckily, they caught

Fat Fact
Recent research indicates that overweight children are more likely to become obese adults.

their problems early and made significant lifestyle changes, literally saving their lives. But it was a real wake-up call for them as to how far they had let themselves go, and they were all humbled by what could have happened had they continued with their unhealthy lifestyles.

I'll admit, I hate going to the doctor as much as the next gal, but you've got to do it. You may not want to go because you're afraid of the news you might hear, but get over it and have a physical done anyhow! Have the physician take your blood pressure and weight, test your reflexes, and draw blood to test for high cholesterol, high blood lipids, diabetes, and other disorders. Tell your doctor any family history you have of cancer, asthma, obesity, heart disease, or other life-threatening illnesses. I know it's scary, but so many diseases can be prevented if they are caught early enough, even cancer. What you don't know could literally kill you.

SUMMARY

You've learned so much about your body in this chapter, your head is probably swimming! Take a few days to think about what you've gotten out of these pages, and come to terms with your genetics, body type, metabolic potential, and overall health status. Recognize who you are and the possibilities afforded you, and you'll be better able to make realistic goals and set out to achieve them with conviction.

HOMEWORK

1. Call your doctor today and make an appointment to get a physical!
2. Look through a bunch of magazines and find three women—celebrity or not—with a body type similar to yours. Notice the clothes they wear, how they accentuate their assets, and try to emulate their confidence.
3. Using the formula on page 12, determine your waist-to-hip ratio. Write it down on the last page of your workout journal under the heading "Results: Week 1." For more information on setting up your workout journal, turn to Chapter 5, page 29.
4. Write down five reasons you want to lose weight and be healthy. They can be anything from keeping up with your kids to running a 5K. Keep this list handy, as you'll revisit it in Chapter 19.
5. Today and for the rest of this week, drink eight full glasses of water. To learn more about the importance of drinking water, turn to page 197.

Extra Credit

Get your body fat checked! Go to a gym that offers skin-fold testing or to a facility with hydrostatic weighing and test yourself. At the end of twelve weeks, return to that facility and get retested.

CHAPTER 3

Your Mind

It's easy to be fat," Suzy from season two of *The Biggest Loser* said to me once at a press junket. In some ways, she's right. It is easy to stay in a familiar place, to maintain the same routine day after day, to do what you've been doing for months or years, to stay within your comfort zone, immune to uncertainty and potential failure.

But is it worth it? Not according to Pam. Pam's parents divorced when she was very young, and she turned to food for comfort. Because of this destructive relationship with food, Pam weighed 140 pounds by the fourth grade. Even though in high school she played volleyball, basketball, and softball, her high activity level did not compensate for the calories she was eating. Pam noticed she was bigger than other girls, and it was harder for her to find a prom dress or buy cute clothes, but she had an outgoing personality and lots of friends. She was OK with being bigger and never tried to diet or lose weight. At her high school graduation, Pam weighed 200 pounds.

Pam played softball in college, but not volleyball or basketball. She essentially cut her activity level in half but didn't adjust her eating habits. Within a few months, Pam had gained an additional 20 pounds. Now, for the first time in her life, she was feeling less OK with her size. She became self-conscious and doubted herself.

Pam had never dieted before, but she became obsessed with getting back below 200 pounds and decided to go on the Atkins diet, a high-protein, high-fat, no-carb eating plan. After several months of struggling, she made it to 197 pounds. Thankful to be done with the restrictive diet, she returned immediately to her old eating habits and within six months had gained back all 23 pounds she had lost, as well as an additional 20, bringing her to an all-time high of 240 pounds. She was crushed! Since Pam had never tried to diet before and had now failed on her very first attempt, her confidence and self-esteem plummeted. She saw herself as a failure.

Pam then gave birth to two children back to back, and while these babies were the light of her life, her weight topped out at 250 pounds and she was ashamed of herself. Pam's outgoing and fun personality crumbled. She was angry and moody, and she frequently yelled at her husband and kids. She knew she was lashing out because she was angry with herself, but she just couldn't control her outbursts. Pam gave up on losing weight and being healthy, and moreover, she gave up on herself. She lost all her self-confidence and spark, and though she put up a good front, behind the scenes she was at rock bottom—depressed, disappointed, and alone.

The day before her daughter's first birthday, Pam was stewing about herself and her weight. How had she let herself get to this point? Then she had an epiphany: She was being incredibly selfish! How could she allow herself to be so unhealthy when she had two little kids depending on her? She decided that she wanted and needed to be able to play with them, tuck them in at night, and walk them down the aisle at their weddings, and that she was done being fat. A fire was lit inside of her; she felt unstoppable. She gave up her feelings of guilt, replaced them with determination, and committed to a health and fitness program that very day. For her, it wasn't easier to be fat. Being fat was destroying her relationships, her marriage, and her personality. She was done with it.

Determination aside, Pam had her work cut out for her, because unfortunately it's not easy *not* to be fat. Every day is a mental struggle, especially in the beginning, and some days it will be all you can do to talk yourself into doing a workout or convince yourself to eat carrot sticks instead of a fast-food burger. Often, the physical work becomes the easy part of the equation, while the mental part becomes more challenging. The good news is that it gets easier! As your new healthy lifestyle becomes a habit, and you begin to see the results of your hard work paying off, things that seemed impossible in the beginning now become routine.

HABITS: MAKE 'EM AND BREAK 'EM

A habit is a regular tendency or addictive practice that is difficult to give up. Sounds serious, huh? Sometimes it is. Some habits are good, such as exercising every morning at 6 a.m. Other habits are bad, such as having fast-food takeout every night for dinner. The trick is to identify the bad habits that are keeping you from achieving a healthy lifestyle and eliminate them while nurturing the good habits you've already established. But breaking a habit is not something that happens overnight. It takes work and conscious attention, but it can and will happen if you want it to.

Many people struggle with emotional eating, using food to fill an unmet emotional need. And it doesn't matter if the emotion is a positive one or a negative one; people get into the habit of eating regardless of the tone of the emotion. This was Karen's problem. Every time she felt an emotion, she found herself in front of the fridge. Let's follow her steps to see how she broke this habit.

- **Recognition.** Every time she was mad, happy, depressed, annoyed, elated, or sad, Karen found herself in the kitchen rooting around for something to eat. Once she recognized this was a habit, Karen noted her mood every time she went to the refrigerator, especially when it was emotionally driven.
- **Question your motives.** Before she opened a bag of chips or pint of ice cream, Karen stopped herself and questioned her motives: Am I really hungry, or is something else driving me to eat a box of cookies?

- **Divert your attention.** Once she stopped herself from eating, Karen would then do something completely different and unrelated to food to break her pattern. She would take her kids out for a bike ride, read a magazine, or clean out the garage. Anything different and unrelated to food was appropriate.
- **Confide in others.** Once she recognized her pattern of emotional eating, Karen confided the habit to her husband. She asked him to help her break the pattern and to call her out when he noticed her falling back into her old ways. This support system helped Karen stick to her intention, and she was able to successfully break her pattern of emotional eating.

Establishing a Habit

Breaking bad habits is only half the story; creating good habits is the other half. Experts say that if you can maintain a behavior for twenty-one to thirty consecutive days, it will become a habit. In theory that doesn't sound like a long time, but on day fourteen, when your alarm goes off at 7 a.m. and it's raining outside and the last thing you want to do is get up and go running, thirty days sounds like an impossible eternity! But if you can just stick with it and follow through with your plan of action, you'll feel better physically and emotionally. And as you repeat the behavior consistently, it really does get easier, I promise! I use these steps with my clients to help them establish a new habit.

- **Choose a habit.** Let's take working out in the morning before work as an example. Formulate an intention to get up at 7 a.m. four days a week to work out. Write this intention down and say it out loud to yourself to make it more real.

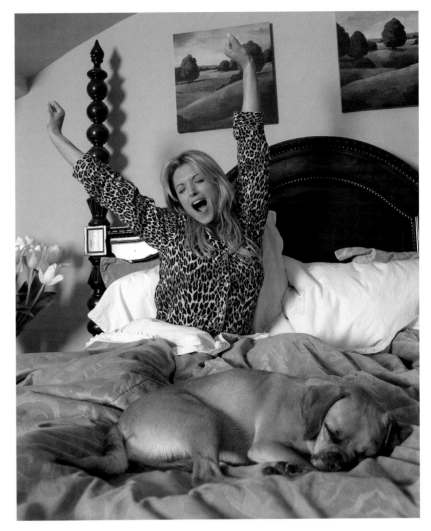

Make a habit of getting up and working out early!

- **Focus on one habit at a time.** Many people try to change all their habits at once. This is simply overwhelming, and chances are you'll end up failing to establish any habits at all. Give one habit your full attention, then move on to others.
- **Take actual steps to make that habit a concrete reality.** No more theorizing about "wanting" or "planning" to work out; now it's time to do it! Set your alarm for 7 a.m. and get up! As an extra incentive, put out your workout clothes the night before, fill your water bottle, and

CLIENT CORNER

JUST SHUT UP AND TRY IT, BY KEN

When I first started training with Kim, I was the king of making excuses for my weight. I had high blood pressure, asthma, sleep apnea, back pain, and arthritis, and I used these ailments to avoid working out. I always had an excuse handy, whether it was exhaustion, pain, or shortness of breath, and I successfully avoided dealing with my weight for years by hiding behind these problems. "I can't" was the staple phrase in my vocabulary. I didn't have faith in my body anymore and was afraid I would hurt myself or, worse, that I wouldn't be able to do what she was asking of me.

Kim finally got fed up with my excuses; she knew I was capable of doing more. So one day when we were working out, she asked me to do squats, and I said, "I can't." Instead of trying to coax me nicely into doing the move like she would normally, this time she got mad and said, "Just shut up and try it." I was so surprised that I did try it, and lo and behold, I did it! And not only did I do it, but it didn't hurt!

All this time I had let my fears direct my life. I had been dealing with injuries for so long and had put up so many mental walls that I had convinced myself that I was capable of far less than I was. Now "Just shut up and try it" is my mantra. I use it on my friends who are just starting to work out or family members who look at my new healthy food with a critical eye. I go into every workout with a positive attitude and back it up with willpower and discipline. And whenever Kim tells me to do something new, I just shut up and try it.

do anything else that makes the process as smooth as possible.

- **Tell someone your intentions.** Inform your spouse or best friend about your plan to work out every day at 7 a.m. and ask that person to check up on you. The more support you can get from friends, family, and work colleagues, the more likely you'll succeed.
- **Stick to it no matter what!** Yes, some days you'll be tired, and that snooze button is super-tempting, but in less than a month you could make working out at 7 a.m. a habit. Isn't that worth the effort?

NEGATIVE SELF-TALK

While Karen's habit of emotional eating was relatively easy to identify, others are not so obvious. One bad habit I notice a lot in my clients is negative self-talk. Many times they don't even realize how they sound, but when they speak about themselves, their goals, and their bodies, it sounds like they are defeated before they even begin. For example, consider these monologues. Which person do you think will succeed with weight loss?

- **Jack:** I really want to start a workout program, but I have a bum knee and the doctor said I can't do lunges. It also hurts when I run or jump a lot. So I want to do something; I just don't know what I can do. My body is falling apart.
- **Sarah:** I'd really like to have a body like Paris Hilton. She's so lean and thin, and my legs are so thick and chunky. I want to work out so I can look like that!
- **Melody:** Everyone in my family is overweight, so it's genetic for me to be fat.

So which one of these people will succeed at weight loss? Surprise! None of them will succeed. Jack is making excuses, enumerating the reasons he can't work out. The more reasons he can come up with, the less likely he will be to start and stick to a healthy lifestyle. Even though he says he "wants" to work out, mentally Jack is not yet ready to make the commitment to change.

Sarah is giving herself an unrealistic role model. As we discussed in Chapter 2, everyone has different body types, and chances are that Sarah's body type is nothing like Paris Hilton's, and no amount of lunges in the world is going to make her legs match those of the hotel heiress. She is setting herself up for disappointment and failure and will probably quit working out when she does not see the unrealistic results she is looking for.

Melody is not accepting responsibility for her own weight and is using genetics as a crutch for her misery. She is blaming her weight problem on uncontrollable circumstances and is resigned to failure before she even begins.

Many times, such negative self-talk is an offshoot of low self-esteem and a lack of self-confidence, and if it's repeated enough, it can become habitual. But really, there is nothing more unattractive than people who are continually putting themselves down, making self-deprecating comments about their bodies, their abilities, and their personalities. People like this come across as weak, depressive, and moody, personality traits that can affect their friendships, relationships, and even their career advancement.

It's to your benefit to learn to speak positively and actively. Speech is a very powerful tool, and the words that come out of your mouth can actually shape your intentions. Learn how to speak in the present, and say "I am" and "I do" instead of "I want" or "I will." And whatever you do, never, *ever* say the word "can't." This is a huge no-no. Unless you're chained to a tree on the side of a cliff and your feet have been cut off at the ankle, you *can* do squats and you *can* do lunges! Even my medically challenged clients have surprised themselves with what they can do when they put their minds to it. Tell yourself you can do it, and it's more than likely you will!

Word Play

Trade negative words and phrases for positive ones!

Negative	Positive
Can't	Can
Won't	Will
Uncontrollable	Manageable
I should	I decide
Weak	Powerful
I wish	I am
Incapable	Able
I'm tired	I'm excited
Don't forget	Remember

MANTRAS

A mantra is a saying you repeat to yourself to encourage a positive response. I know; this sounds like some touchy-feely yoga gig, and it kind of is. But the good news is that your mantra can be whatever floats your boat. It doesn't have to be some sort of weird medieval chanting noise or an obnoxious breathing exercise. It can be anything you want that empowers and motivates you to push through the pain and achieve your goal. For instance, one of my clients would say, "Go, dog, go!" to pump out those last few reps of an exercise when he was feeling tired. At first I laughed and asked him what that was all about. He explained that he was reading *Go, Dog, Go!* by P. D. Eastman to his kids every night—it was their favorite book.

SUMMARY

The mental side of losing weight is often more difficult than the physical side, and in the coming weeks you might struggle more with your mental roadblocks than with anything else. Whether you've tried a diet and failed like Pam or make excuses why you can't work out like Ken, these cerebral hang-ups and habits can be overcome. Practice identifying your mental barriers and dedicate some time to breaking them down one by one. The more barriers you break down, the better you'll feel about yourself and the whole weight-loss process, and the more likely you'll be to succeed!

HOMEWORK

1. Write down a list of bad habits that are keeping you from reaching your goals. Now use the steps on pages 16–18 to help guide you in breaking those habits and establishing good ones instead.

2. Listen to yourself speak for one whole day. Mentally note or physically write down how many times you criticize yourself or others, say the word "can't," or make an excuse. The following day, make a conscious effort to speak positively and actively.

3. Come up with a mantra to use during intense cardio and resistance-training work, and say it out loud three times. Come up with another mantra to use during flexibility training and cooling-down periods, and say it out loud three times.

4. Today and for the rest of this week, trade simple carbohydrates such as bread, pasta, and fruit juice for complex carbohydrates such as brown rice, yams, and oatmeal. To read more about complex carbohydrates and their role in weight loss, turn to page 192.

Saying "Go, dog, go!" to himself helped remind him why he was here working out in the first place—so he could lose weight and be around later in life to see his kids grow up.

   Try out a few different mantras and see what resonates with who you are and what your intention is. I like to choose different ones according to my activity at the time. If I am relaxing and stretching, for instance, I use a soothing saying such as "I am unwinding and regenerating." If I am running stairs, however, I might use a song lyric with a good, solid beat to keep my mental energy high.

CHAPTER 4

Your Goals

Nothing feels better than reaching a goal. We've all experienced this feeling, whether you worked hard and got a promotion, or trained hard and ran a 10K. Setting and reaching goals is incredibly motivating, and nothing encourages weight-loss adherence more than this simple procedure. Your goals will change as your fitness level changes, and chances are you'll underestimate yourself and what you can accomplish at first. But once you start to make progress, see results, and one by one reach your short- and long-term goals, you'll be more motivated and self-confident and excited to set more goals. Eventually, you'll learn to set the bar high enough to challenge yourself but not so high that you set yourself up for failure.

GET-REAL QUESTIONS

I want you to be able to achieve any and all goals you set for yourself, whether they're as simple as eating more vegetables or as lofty as running a marathon. To ensure you achieve what you intend, you've got to get real about yourself and your life. The more honest you are about the time you have to spend on your fitness

program, the more likely you will be to set and reach some realistic goals. Consider these questions:

- How many days per week are you able to commit to your workout program?
- How much time per day are you able to commit to your workout program?
- Do you travel a lot for work?
- Do you have a family and/or a spouse?
- What activities do you like to do?
- What activities would you like to do in the future?
- Do you have any health problems, injuries, or physical limitations?

How Many Days per Week Are You Able to Commit to Your Workout Program?

Most people set themselves up for failure because they expect too much of themselves and are disappointed when they fail. But if you're busy with work, family, and social activities, you're not going to have time to work out seven days a week. Heck, you might not even get in four days a week—and that's OK. Create goals that work with your life and the time you have instead of expecting the impossible. That

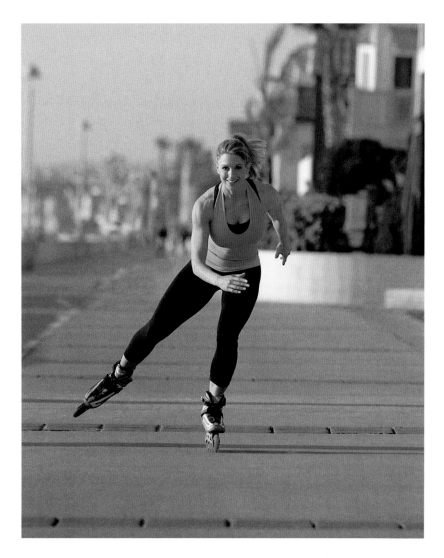

you can split it up. Do half an hour in the morning or at lunch and another half an hour in the evening, or split your workout into three 20-minute sessions throughout the day. Look at your schedule and fit it in. There is always time—you just have to make it!

Do You Travel a Lot for Work?

Travel is exhausting—long hours on planes, time changes, poor food choices, and dehydration, but you can stick to your goals and stay fit while on the road with a little planning. Book a hotel that has a health club, join a gym with nationwide locations, or pack a set of fitness bands in your suitcase to work out in your room. Also, be mindful of your food choices while traveling to stay on track. Make your goals realistic, but also make fitness a priority no matter whether you're in your living room suite or the Embassy Suites.

Do You Have a Family and/or a Spouse?

Many people feel guilty or selfish when they begin a workout plan because they think they are taking time away from their family or spouse. But truthfully, a healthy parent or spouse is a better parent or spouse, so instead of looking at your family as adversaries, look at them as supporters. Tell them about your goals and intentions, and ask them to support you in your decision to live a healthier life. Some of them might even like to join you in your new program, and voilà—you've got instant workout buddies!

What Activities Do You Like to Do?

You're more likely to stick to your workout goals if you're doing something you like. For instance, I am not a runner—I don't like it, never have, and never will! But I love to in-line skate. Therefore, it's smarter

Bright Idea
To make sure you get your workout in while traveling, change your clothes as soon as you get to your hotel, and immediately go to the hotel gym to work out or take a jog around the neighborhood.

way, when you fulfill—or even exceed!—those goals, you feel accomplished instead of let down.

How Much Time per Day Are You Able to Commit to Your Workout Program?

You don't need to work out three hours a day to get results. In fact, this can lead to overtraining, boredom, and burnout. An hour a day is all you really need to make healthy, physical gains that can change your life. Ideally, try to do the workout all at once, but if you're extremely busy, for me to skate than it is to force myself to run. Try a bunch of different activities and see what you enjoy best. Yoga, kickboxing, Spinning, and other group fitness classes are great ways to enjoy cardio exercise.

What Activities Would You Like to Do in the Future?

For instance, running a 10K or planning a ski vacation are great incentives to get in shape. Even if you've never done anything similar before, that does not mean you can't do it now! Decide you're going to do it, then map out a plan of action. Aim high, but chart your course wisely.

Do You Have Any Health Problems, Injuries, or Physical Limitations?

If so, first get the go-ahead from your physician and follow any guidelines the doctor suggests when planning your fitness program. Next, stop making excuses! Health problems are not a reason to slack off. In fact, exercising and eating right can reverse problems such as diabetes, arthritis, back pain, stress, even depression. Of course, be mindful of your injuries and limitations so as not to exacerbate your problems; create goals that take your injuries and limitations into account but that still challenge you within healthy boundaries.

MAKING GOALS

Now that you've considered all those questions, it's time to get busy making goals! You're going to make one large long-term goal to be reached at the end of the twelve-week *Your Body, Your Life* program and several short-term goals to help move you toward that long-term goal successfully. Your goals should all be attainable, realistic, and reasonable. For example, losing 50 pounds in a month for your

high school reunion is not a reasonable goal and will ultimately lead to failure. But planning to lose weight steadily at a rate of 1 or 2 pounds a week over the course of several months offers a better chance of success.

Long-Term Goals

Your long-term goal is the big kahuna, the light at the end of the time tunnel, the tree house at the top of the ladder. This is the ultimate goal you're shooting for in the next twelve weeks. But even though this goal is akin to the brass ring on the carousel, try not to make it overwhelming. For instance, a novice runner will never be able to run a marathon with only two months of training. It's impossible! But if that same runner decides to run a marathon at the end of twelve months, he or she is very likely to succeed.

Make your long-term goal as concrete as possible. You should be able to envision yourself at the end of the process, happy, successful, and accomplished. For example, here is an abstract goal my client Marilyn made last New Year's:

> *"I will adopt a healthy lifestyle in the coming year."*

The sentiment is correct, but there is no "action" to this statement, nothing concrete for Marilyn to build on. Moreover, it's not exciting, and neither one of us was jazzed up when she said it out loud. So we worked on it a while and came up with this revised version:

> *"In the next year, I will work out three to five times a week and will focus on eating healthy, wholesome foods to achieve a weight loss of 1 to 2 pounds per week. Within the next twelve*

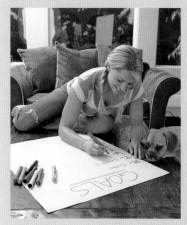
months, I aim to lose at least 50 pounds and regain my endurance and energy."

Now, that's a goal! Unlike her first statement, this goal outlines several concrete steps Marilyn could see in her mind's eye that would guide her toward achieving this goal. When she read it out loud, Marilyn got excited. She could imagine the process with this statement and was eager to begin that day.

Examples of Great Long-Term Goals
- **Margie:** I will complete all twelve weeks of the *Your Body, Your Life* program, getting up an hour earlier to exercise before work four to five days a week. By this summer I will lose 10 pounds, will look great in a bikini, and will celebrate by taking a trip to Hawaii with my family!
- **Sally:** I will lose 10 to 12 pounds in three months by exercising four days a week. I will cook more healthy meals for myself and my fiancé so that by my wedding date (in three months and one week!), I will fit into my original size 8 wedding dress and won't have to pay for massive alterations!
- **Kate:** In the next twelve weeks, I will eat healthy and exercise regularly to get my diabetes under control. I intend to be medication free by this time next year.

Seal the Deal

It's important to write your long-term goal in your workout journal so you can refer to it regularly and remind yourself of your intentions. On the very first page or inside cover of your workout journal, write your long-term goal in big, bold letters. You can even get crazy with yourself and decorate it with stickers, colored markers, pictures, or other fun things. For instance, last February my goal was to get in shape for a trip I was taking to Hawaii, and I cut out pictures of palm trees, sunblock lotions, bikinis, and dolphins from magazines and stuck them all over my goal page. Every time I looked at it, I remembered my end goal and was more determined than ever to reach it!

Short-Term Goals

Short-term goals are like the rungs on the ladder that enable you to reach that long-term goal at the top. Like your long-term goal, each smaller goal should be concrete and imaginable, helping map out a progression of achievement. I like to break short-term goals into categories: monthly, weekly, and daily.

Monthly Goals

At the beginning of each month, decide what your monthly goal will be. Write this goal in your journal and refer to it often to keep you on course. At the end of the month, revisit this goal and decide whether you have achieved it.

Examples of Good Monthly Goals
- I will lose up to 6 pounds this month with good nutrition and exercise.
- I will master the Level I *Your Body, Your Life* circuits.
- I will cook more for my family, ordering healthy takeout no more than once a week.
- I will use my thirty-day trial gym membership to try some group fitness classes.

Weekly Goals

Weekly goals are not as large as monthly goals, so don't go overboard with your expectations. At the beginning of each week, decide what your goal is going to be and write it down in your journal. At the end of the week, revisit this goal and decide whether you've achieved it.

Examples of Good Weekly Goals
- I will eat more green vegetables.
- I will get up an hour earlier three days this week to do my circuits before work.
- I will walk the 1-mile distance from the subway to my office two days this week instead of taking a cab.
- I will use my lunch hour this week to do cardio or stretch instead of doing paperwork that can wait.

Daily Goals

Though daily goals are the smallest in terms of time, they are the biggest in terms of immediate satisfaction. Make your next day's goal right before bed and write it in your journal. It can be anything you think will make you happier, healthier, and more successful with your fitness plan.

Examples of Good Daily Goals
- I will bring my lunch to work tomorrow so I don't order Chinese takeout (again!).
- I will put some chicken in to marinate before leaving for work tomorrow so I can have a healthy dinner when I get home.
- I will resist the urge to have a doughnut at 3 p.m. and instead will bring my own snack of Wasa crackers and peanut butter.
- Tomorrow, I will get up and stretch lightly at least once an hour at work to keep my back from tightening up.

WEIGHT LOSS AS A GOAL

Whenever I ask new clients what they want to achieve with their fitness program, the universal answer is "Weight loss." Many clients end up being thankful for things other than weight loss, such as an increase in energy, an ability to do more and be more active, and a new sense of purpose, but initially everyone wants to lose a few pounds. How do you make weight loss into a realistic goal? Let's do a little math.

One pound of fat is equal to 3,500 stored calories. In order to lose 1 pound of fat, you've got to burn off those additional calories while still maintaining your basal metabolic rate (BMR).

A safe number of pounds to lose is 1 to 2 per week. This number represents actual fat pounds lost, not those lost from water deficit or normal fluctuations in scale weight. In order to lose 1 pound of fat in a week, you've got to create a caloric deficit of 3,500 calories. Sounds like a lot,

TEN 100-CALORIE NIBBLES YOU CAN ELIMINATE *TODAY*!

- 5 Saltine crackers
- 2 slices of bacon
- 2½ Girl Scout Thin Mint cookies
- 1 8-ounce can of Coke
- 1 tablespoon butter
- 25 Jelly Belly Jelly Beans
- ⅔ cup whole milk
- 4 Hershey's Kisses
- 1 ounce regular American cheese
- ½ (8 ounces) Starbucks Tall Blended Mocha Frappucino

TEN ACTIVITIES THAT BURN 100 CALORIES *TODAY*!*

- 60 minutes of grocery shopping
- 20 minutes of athletic sex!
- 30 minutes of playing fetch with your dog
- 30 minutes of gardening
- 30 minutes of washing your car
- 20 minutes of shoveling snow
- 30 minutes of vacuuming
- 20 minutes of stretching
- 60 minutes of cooking dinner and washing the dishes
- 60 minutes of piano playing

Based on a 150-pound woman

Web Watch

For an unbelievable list of activities and the calories they burn, check out www.caloriesperhour.com!

huh? But when you break it down over the course of a week, it's not too bad.

Let's look at Amy. Amy needs to eat 1,400 calories a day to maintain her BMR and keep her metabolism running. Any fewer than that, and she'll put her body in "starvation mode," halting progress and putting her metabolism at risk. (See Chapter 11, "The Bad Fad," for more on this topic!) But Amy currently eats about 1,800 calories a day, 400 more than she needs. If Amy simply cuts back on her daily caloric intake without compromising her BMR requirements, she'll begin to lose weight. This daily 400-calorie deficit adds up to 2,800 calories over the course of a week! Now let's add in exercise three days a week, which burns an estimated 400 calories per workout. In those three days, Amy burns an additional 1,200 calories. Add that to the 2,800 from her

dietary modifications, and she has burned 4,000 calories, more than a pound of fat lost in only a week!

See, it can be done! Just make sure you lose only 1 to 2 pounds of fat per week. If you try to lose more than that, you're losing not fat but rather muscle tissue. I know you may be impatient, but stick to the moderate path and you'll be able to keep that fat off for life.

MOVING GOALS

Another great goal is to incorporate more activity into your daily life. Yes, you still have to exercise to get fit and lose weight! But you'll be surprised how quickly little things can add up to a whole mess of extra calories burned during the course of the day. Every little bit counts.

BURNING QUESTION

What are pedometers? Pedometers are little pager-size gadgets that count steps by sensing motion. Just hook one to your belt or pants and get moving! The pedometer will count your steps no matter whether you're strolling to the bathroom at work or running on the gym treadmill. Pedometers are great for measuring your daily activity level. Wear one for a whole day—from the moment you get up to the moment you go to bed—and record how many steps you take. Write this number in your workout journal. Each day, try to match or increase that amount of steps by adding more activity to your day. Research has shown that taking 10,000 steps a day is equivalent to getting 30 minutes of physical activity. Simple pedometers are cheap (about ten bucks), while more complicated ones that calculate calories burned and other such details can be more pricey (thirty to one hundred dollars).

REWARDS!

Every job well done deserves a reward! The rewards you use for reaching fitness goals should all be healthy and positive. I never recommend rewarding yourself with food or food-related activities. Instead, come up with calorie-free indulgences such as a mani/pedi, some new music for your iPod, even a new pair of workout socks. If you've got a family, get your kids and spouse to participate in your reward so you can all feel great about your accomplishment. Go to the beach for a day, take a family hike, or go to a hockey game. You'll spend quality time with your loved ones while enjoying an active reward for yourself.

My rule of thumb is this: The larger the goal accomplished, the larger the reward! For instance, if you went a whole week without snacking in the break room, reward yourself with a nice, hot bath and have your spouse watch the kids for half an hour. If you reached a bigger goal, such as losing 20 pounds, reward yourself with something more substantial, such as a weekend vacation, a spa day with your friends, even a new outfit to dress up your new stylin' bod! Here are some of the ingenious rewards some of my clients have come up with in the past:

"I finally ran—not walked!—my first 5K after three months of training, and bought myself a top-of-the-line pair of Nike Air Trainers I had been coveting! My poor feet deserve them!"

"When I finally fit back into my favorite size 10 jeans, I bought a great new pair of shoes to wear with those pants and took my boyfriend out dancing!"

"This week I rewarded myself with one new song on iTunes for every time I resisted the doughnuts in the break room at work. Now I'm excited because I have two new playlists for when I do cardio!"

"I lost 40 pounds in six months, reaching my goal weight of 145 pounds! I celebrated with my family by taking a trip we had been talking about for months— we all went to Sea World."

"After a year, I finally reached my goal weight of 150 pounds, and bought myself the best club-quality treadmill money could buy. Yes, it's extravagant, but I'm worth it!"

SUMMARY

Making realistic, attainable goals is an essential part of the weight-loss process. Not only does it move you forward toward your ultimate goal of making fitness a lifestyle, but it also instills a feeling of accomplishment and pride as one by one you reach goal after goal and become healthier and more excited about your new life.

Fun Fact
Thomas Jefferson invented the first pedometer!

TEN WAYS TO BE MORE ACTIVE *TODAY*!

- When traveling, walk around the airport between flights instead of sitting at your gate.
- Take the stairs at work instead of the elevator.
- Park at the farthest end of the parking lot when shopping.
- Instead of e-mailing your co-workers, get up and walk to their desk to chat.
- Wash your own car instead of taking it to the car wash.
- Set an hourly alarm on your computer or Blackberry reminding you to get up and take a lap around the office or the block.
- Use a hand basket instead of a pushcart at the grocery store when purchasing only a few items.
- Take a walk around the block while your chicken or lasagna is baking in the oven.
- Get off the bus or subway early and walk the rest of the way to your destination.
- Go out dancing with your friends instead of going to the movies.

HOMEWORK

1. Using the points made in this chapter, decide on your long-term goal. Use the twelve-week period for the *Your Body, Your Life* program as your time frame. Write your goal in your workout journal.

2. Come up with a really creative reward for reaching your long-term goal!

3. Using the points made in this chapter, decide on your short-term goals as they arise. Begin with the monthly goals, then work your way to the weekly and daily goals.

4. Come up with creative rewards for reaching your short-term goals!

5. Make a goal poster or goal T-shirt! Use the guidelines on page 24 to help you.

6. Today and the rest of this week, eat more fresh fruits and vegetables. To read more about the importance of fresh produce, turn to page 192!

Extra Credit

Go out and buy a pedometer. Over the course of three days, record how many steps you typically take, writing it in your workout journal each time. Then, in coming weeks, try to increase that number of steps by 100–300 each day by incorporating more movement into your daily life, recording your results in your journal. At the end of twelve weeks, compare your beginning number with your ending number. How did you do?

CHAPTER 5

Your Journals

Journals are a great way to stay on track with a fitness program. They keep you accountable to yourself and your goals, and serve as a recorded measure of your successes, setbacks, and ultimate progress. Think of these journals as diaries, but instead of writing down which boy you want to ask you to prom (okay, maybe I am still living in high school!), write down what kind of workout you did, or what sort of food you ate. You're going to have two journals in the *Your Body, Your Life* program: one for workouts and one for food.

WORKOUT JOURNALS

Workout journals make you accountable, and accountability is huge when it comes to sticking to a program. People who are the most successful plan their workouts in advance. This may be tricky sometimes if you're super-busy, but I guarantee that if you look hard enough, you'll find the time to work out. Investigate your schedule a week ahead. See whether you've got business or family obligations, important appointments, or other commitments coming up, then write in your workouts around them so you don't run into any roadblocks. The physical act of writing down your workout turns an abstract idea into a concrete appointment to take care of your body and your health. Breaking this commitment is like breaking a promise to yourself.

Once you've got your days and times mapped out, write down what you plan to do each of those days. Will you do the Level II Trouble Spots Circuit first thing in the morning, or your 30 minutes of cardio after work on Monday? Whatever you choose, inscribe it in your calendar in bold letters.

Take a look at Shelly's workout week (page 30), for example. Usually, Shelly trains after work, but this week she has a series of business meetings, client dinners, and family obligations and has to rearrange her workouts to accommodate her schedule.

Although she is really busy this week, Shelly was still able to schedule in five workouts! She carefully planned her workouts around her other obligations and was able to get them all in, making for a successful week!

Shelly's Workout Schedule

Monday	6:30 a.m. (before work), Level I, Circuit 1
Tuesday	Off—daughter's recital
Wednesday	12:30 p.m. (at lunch), cardio, 20 minutes of walking
Thursday	6:30 a.m. (before work), Level I, Circuit 2
Friday	Off—dinner "date" with husband
Saturday	8 a.m. (before family outing), Level I, Lower Body/Cardio Circuit
Sunday	6 p.m. (after son's softball tournament), Trouble Spots Circuit

Bright Idea

If you have a Palm Pilot or Blackberry, set an alarm to remind you of your workout that day!

Note to Self

Write your workouts in pencil! That way if a catastrophe occurs, you can easily move your workout to the next day.

BURNING QUESTION

I want to work out regularly, but I can't find the time. What should I do? There is no such thing as "finding the time" to do anything. You have to make the time. Look objectively at your schedule and see where exercise can fit in. Do you have time while your baby naps? How about early in the morning before work? If you're extremely busy, you'll probably have to get creative with your scheduling. Also, look objectively at your lifestyle. Many people waste time doing things such as watching TV, playing computer games, even talking on the phone, when they could be working out instead. Once you stop making excuses and make fitness a priority, you'll miraculously "find" the time needed to work out and will be happier and healthier for it.

Workout Notes

After each workout, write in your journal about how it went. Anything you can note

about the workout, your feelings, and your energy level will be useful in the future. Over time, patterns will emerge that will help you refine or change your program according to the results you're getting. For each workout journal entry, consider these questions:

- **What time did you work out?** Was it the time you had intended? Why or why not?
- **How did you feel before and after the workout?** Did it help you unwind? Did it fire you up? Did it make you tired or energized? Did it help you shake off the day and refocus?
- **What did you do and for how long?** Did you do cardio or a circuit? What exercises did you do and at what level? Was any particular exercise hard/easy for you? How long did you do your circuits for?
- **Anything else?** Were you stressed from work? PMS-ing? Did you have a fight with your boyfriend the night before? Were you excited about an upcoming date?

Managing the Detours

Sometimes, even the best-laid plans are derailed—the kids get sick, your car breaks down, or, like Gina, you have to stay late at work to finish a project (see page 31). But guess what—it's not the end of the world! It's within your power to reschedule that workout for a different day or time. Many people have this all-or-nothing mentality—*If I can't stick to my plan exactly as written, I may as well stuff it and go back to my old ways!* But if you miss a workout, don't freak! Just open your journal, look at your schedule, and redraw the plans. Schedule the workout for the next day, or use the day you missed

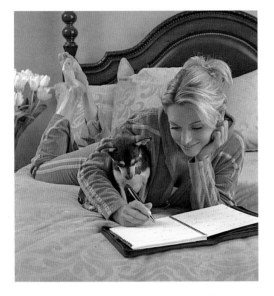

as an "off" day. It's OK to move things around; just get your workouts in when you can manage.

FOOD JOURNALS

Food journals are private, recorded logs detailing exactly what you put in your mouth and when. They keep you accountable for your food intake and can highlight patterns of emotional eating, indicate missing or excessive food groups, and help you better formulate a healthy eating plan to help you lose weight and keep it off.

I always, always recommend food journals to my clients, especially those beginning or restarting a fitness program after a long hiatus. I can safely say that no one accurately tells me—or themselves!—the truth about how many calories they are eating. Whether they choose to delude themselves deliberately or are embarrassed to admit their poor eating habits, I typically find a 500–2,000-calorie difference in the recorded calories eaten versus the admitted calories eaten! That's a lot!

For this reason, I recommend keeping a food log for a full week before changing

Sample Workout Journal Entry: Gina

Monday	Off		
Tuesday	8 p.m.	Circuit 1	Felt really tired when I started, but eventually shook it off and felt pretty good when I was done. Got through my full 30 seconds of squats today—yay! First time so far.
Wednesday	6 p.m.	Cardio	Did my cardio for the week—25 minutes of power walking. Mike bailed out on me so I had to fly solo. Was OK—listened to my new playlist.
Thursday	Agh!	Missed	Was supposed to do the Lower Body/Cardio workout today but had to stay late at work. Will double up and do it tomorrow with the Trouble Spots workout. Oh, well. *C'est la vie!*
Friday	7 p.m.	Lower Body/ Cardio and Trouble Spots	Did Trouble Spots first, then Lower Body/Cardio. Really felt it in my glutes today! Am very tired, though. Think I might be PMS-ing. All I want is chocolate chip cookies.
Saturday	10 a.m.	Circuit 2	I kicked butt! Got a lot of sleep, had an extra cup of coffee, and killed that workout. I think I can see some shoulder muscles forming! That makes me feel pretty good.
Sunday	10 a.m.	Cardio	Felt great and energetic this morning, so I did an extra 20 minutes of cardio this week. Went power walking around the neighborhood.

Sample Food Journal Entry:
Two Days in the Life of Debby—Day 1

Monday	6 a.m.	*Breakfast:* 6 egg whites, 1 slice wheat toast with 1 tbsp peanut butter, 1 cup coffee with 1 packet Splenda, 1 glass water, vitamin. *Comments:* Tired this morning and sluggish. Grabbed another cup of coffee on the way to work. Had real sugar in it, two packs! Oops.
	??	*Snack:* Missed because of meetings
	2 p.m.	*Lunch:* Cafeteria lasagna with slice of French garlic bread (with butter!), 1 Diet Coke. *Comments:* Felt extremely guilty eating this, but was starving and ate the whole thing. Ate lunch late because of work meetings. Am way over my fat calories for the day already. The Diet Coke seems ironic . . .
	4:30 p.m.	*Snack:* 1 large apple, 2 low-fat string cheeses, 1 large bottle water. *Comments:* Shouldn't really be eating cheese again since I had so much at lunch, but it was all I brought. Didn't want to have a doughnut as a snack.
	8 p.m.	*Dinner:* 6 ounces tuna mixed with 2 tbsp mayo and 1 tsp mustard. Eaten on 1 toasted slice of wheat bread. 1 small mixed green salad with 1 tbsp low-fat vinaigrette dressing. *Comments:* I did extra cardio after my workout to try to counterbalance the fat I ate at lunch, but think the day is a wash. *Tomorrow's goal:* Try to eat on a more regular schedule.

anything about your eating habits. This log can help identify patterns, habits, and other quirks you may have regarding food and give you a good idea of what you need to do to change those habits for the better. Write down anything and everything you eat or drink during this week, whether it's an entire meal, a piece of gum, or a single Hershey's Kiss. And be honest! There is no point in lying to yourself about what you're eating. No one will know your tally but you.

At the end of the week, add up how many calories you took in each day using a simple calorie-counting book or online service—I think you'll be surprised! The little nibbles here and there really add up, as do high-calorie drinks such as soda, sugary coffees, and juices. With a week's worth of eaten food laid out in front of you, you'll be able to see where you can cut out snacking, emotional eating, and excessive drinking, and you'll have a good handle on what you need to do to lose weight.

Food Notes

Once you've completed your weekly food log, you're ready to start with your regular food journal. After each meal or snack—intended or happenstance!—write about it in your journal. These entries don't have to be essays, delving into the darkest recesses of your brain! They can be one word or a sentence that accurately relates important information about that meal. For each food journal entry, consider these questions:

• What time did you eat?
• What did you eat?
• How much of it did you have?
• How much water did you drink? What else did you drink, and how much?
• How did you feel before eating? How did you feel after eating?

• Are you having any cravings?
• Did you take a vitamin?

Managing the Detours

Expecting to eat perfectly every single day is not realistic, because things happen. Maybe you sleep through your alarm like Debby and miss breakfast, or maybe you have a long work meeting that runs through your lunch hour. If you are off schedule with your eating or are bummed that you ate something you shouldn't have eaten, don't let it completely ruin your day. Again, many people have that all-or-nothing attitude and think, *I ate a big brownie and ruined my diet; why not eat the whole pan? The day is a mess already anyhow!* But if you have a treat or fall off the food wagon, don't freak out! Try to eat clean the rest of the day, and resolve to stay on track the next day. Make daily short-term goals that reinforce these resolutions like Debby did, like planning to drink more water or to eat on a more regular schedule, and don't beat yourself up if you have a weak moment or two. If you have a cupcake once a month for a birthday party, it's absolutely not the end of the world! Life is for living, and food is to be enjoyed; just enjoy it in small, controlled quantities and you'll be fine.

SUMMARY

Journals can be wonderful tools when you're trying to lose weight and change your lifestyle. They make you accountable for your workouts and eating habits and can help identify good and bad patterns that can inhibit or accelerate your progress. The more detailed and honest you are with your journal entries, the more they will benefit you now and in the future.

Sample Food Journal Entry: Two Days in the Life of Debby—Day 2

Tuesday	7 a.m.	*Breakfast:* 1 apple, coffee with 1 packet Splenda in thermos. *Comments:* Got up late and ran out the door! Packed two good snacks for work last night; will eat one as breakfast when I get to the office.
	8:15 a.m.	*Snack:* Small baggie of raw almonds, 3 large celery sticks. *Comments:* Traffic! Couldn't wait until I got to work. Ate my first snack in the car. So much for eating on schedule.
	10 a.m.	*Snack:* ½ turkey sandwich I brought for lunch, 1 large bottle of water. *Comments:* Skipping breakfast sucks! I am hungry no matter what I eat today!
	11 a.m.	1 birthday cupcake *Comments:* It's Ann-Marie's birthday and they were my favorite—vanilla with chocolate icing!
	1 p.m.	*Lunch:* ½ turkey sandwich, 1 Diet Coke
	3 p.m.	1 Diet Coke *Comments:* I am craving sugar . . . hopefully this will do as a substitute.
	4 p.m.	*Snack:* 2 Wasa crackers with hummus, water.
	8 p.m.	*Dinner:* Homemade turkey meatballs with ¼ cup red sauce, large green salad with non-fat dressing, 1 glass red wine. *Comments:* What a rotten day of eating! But instead of having sugary treats, I had a Diet Coke, which was good. If I am late again, I vow to take three minutes and make a smoothie for breakfast so I'm not starving. *Tomorrow's goal:* Didn't drink enough water, so tomorrow I will focus on that!

HOMEWORK

1. If you haven't already, buy two journals, one for your workouts and one for your food.
2. Sit down with your social and work schedules and objectively find the time four to five days a week to work out.
3. Keep a food log for one whole week, marking down anything and everything that passes your lips. At the end of the week, analyze your entries, and identify any patterns that may emerge, such as emotional eating, bingeing, or infrequent mealtimes.
4. Today and the rest of this week, incorporate more fiber into your daily diet. For more information on the importance of fiber, turn to page 196!

CHAPTER 6

Your Fitness

Once upon a time, Janet was a track athlete, a hurdler, in fact. She was all-state in high school and even competed at the collegiate level for a few years. After college, she got married, took a job, had a family, and, aside from an occasional jog around the 'hood with the stroller, all but abandoned track and field. After giving birth to her third son, Janet came to me for personal training. Although she hadn't worked out seriously in nearly eight years, Janet still considered herself a highly trained athlete. She explained to me the type of program she was expecting, one she remembered from her days as a collegiate hurdler: It involved very heavy lifting in the gym and some serious cardiovascular work, including sprint drills, 50-yard dashes and stair work. It exhausted me just thinking about it, but Janet was unfazed—she fully believed she could handle this program because in her mind, she was still that collegiate hurdler; she did not realize how out of shape she really was—until she took my standard fitness test.

Janet was shocked. Her endurance and strength were poor at best, and her flexibility was minimal. At first she was depressed. How had she let herself get so out of shape? Track had been her whole life; she had been a powerful, elite athlete and she had let that talent slip through her fingers! But then she remembered her wonderful family, her three sons, and the terrific life she now led. Things were different now; she was different; her priorities were different. She lifted her chin, set her jaw, and quickly got over it. She wrote her fitness test results in red pen on a large piece of paper and taped it to her fridge between her sons' drawings and report cards. Every day she looked at that paper and reminded herself of her intentions to improve, steeling her resolve. At the gym she got stronger and faster and more flexible, working hard to improve her fitness and her body. Today, Janet is in her best shape since college. While she may not be leaping any track hurdles tomorrow, she successfully cleared her huge inactivity hurdle and is now sprinting toward her fitness finish line!

Like Janet, you need to know your starting point before beginning a fitness program. Some people tend to overdo it, especially if they were athletic previously, while others simply don't know their capabilities. In this chapter, you'll be taking your measurements, testing your physical fitness, and weighing yourself. Believe me, I know this is going to be super-hard! But as disappointing as these numbers may be at first, remember that this is the last time you'll weigh this much or will be this many inches around the waist or hips. Think of these measurements as the starting blocks on a track; once you push off and start running, you'll never see them again! So take a deep breath, and just do it.

YOUR MEASUREMENTS

Using a soft cloth measuring tape, measure around your waist, hips, thigh, and upper arm. Use the photographs below to guide you on the tape placement. Write your measurements in the back of your workout journal under the heading "Results Week 1" or on a piece of paper you can keep handy. At the end of twelve weeks, you'll retake these measurements and will compare your end results with your starting point. I guarantee you'll be pleased with your progress!

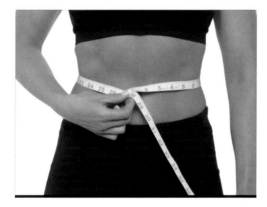

Waist: Measure at the smallest part between the hips and the rib cage.

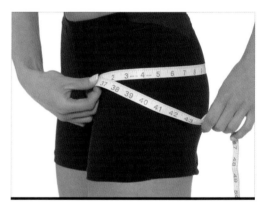

Hips: Measure around the largest part of your lower body. (Yes, that means your butt!)

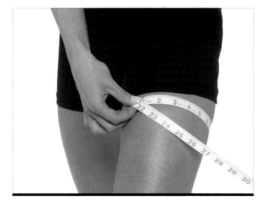

Thigh: Measure the widest part on both legs.

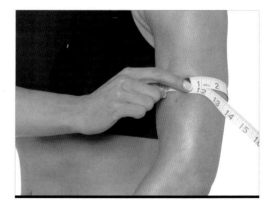

Upper arm: Measure halfway between the elbow and the shoulder on both arms.

YOUR PHYSICAL FITNESS

Take these simple fitness tests to get an idea of your current strength, endurance, and flexibility levels. Record your results underneath your measurements on your workout journal results page or on your paper. In twelve weeks, retake this test and compare your results. You'll be astounded with your progress!

Push-up Test

Tests: Upper-body strength and endurance

Instructions: Do as many push-ups as you can in 1 minute using good form.

Kneel on the floor and place your hands on the ground outside your shoulders. Balance your weight between your hands and your knees, keeping your torso rigid and your abs tight. Bend your elbows to lower your torso almost to the floor, then press back up to the start ("up") position.*

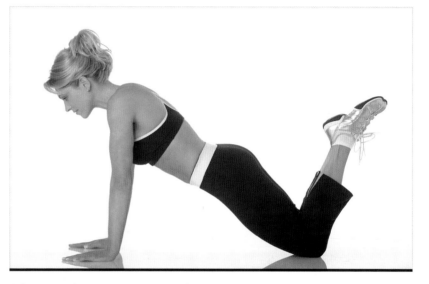

*If you need to rest at any point during this test, rest in the "up" position.

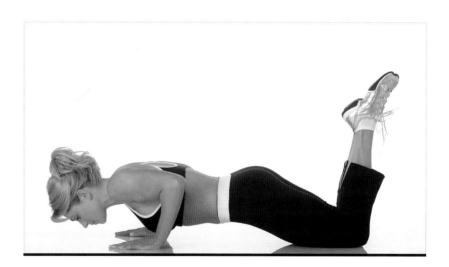

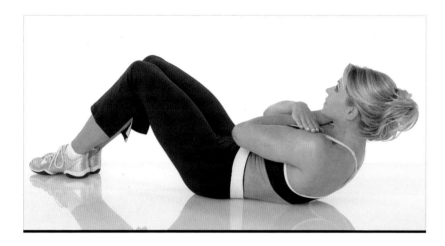

Crunch Test

Tests: Abdominal strength and endurance

Instructions: Do as many crunches as you can in 1 minute using good form.

Lie on your back with your arms crossed over your chest, your knees bent, and your feet flat on the floor. Lift your chin off your chest and focus on a point on the ceiling. Exhale and slowly lift your head, shoulders, and upper back off the floor. Slowly lower to the start and repeat right away.

Squat Test

Tests: Lower-body strength and endurance

Instructions: Do as many squats as you can in 1 minute with good form.

Stand with your feet hip-width apart and your hands on your hips. Slowly squat toward the floor, bending your knees and kicking your hips back as if you were going to sit in a chair. When your thighs are almost parallel to the floor, or your heels begin to lift, stand back up to the start position.

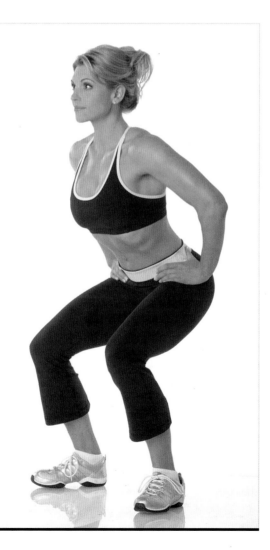

Sit-and-Reach Test

Tests: Hamstring and lower-back flexibility

Instructions: Repeat this test three times through, taking the best of the three results.

Lay a yardstick on the floor and tape it down with a perpendicular piece of masking tape. Sit on the floor by the zero end of the stick, and extend your legs to either side. Line your heels up with the 15-inch mark, feet flexed, and legs spaced about 12 inches apart. Place one hand on top of the other and slowly lean forward as far as you can, gliding your fingertips along the yardstick. Don't bounce or force the stretch; simply exhale and lean forward as far as you can while keeping your knees straight. Note the number your fingertips reach on the yard-stick. Sit up, rest a moment, and try again. Repeat three times.

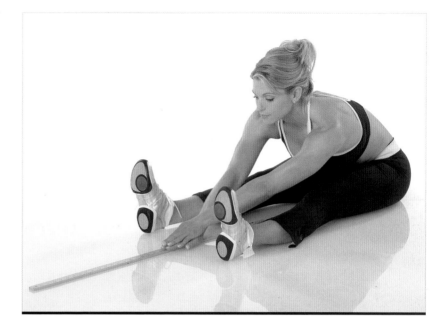

Finger-Touch Test

Tests: Shoulder flexibility

Instructions: Do this test on both sides, as your two arms may not have the same range of motion.

Lift your right arm straight up overhead close to your ear, and bend your elbow so your right hand falls between your shoulder blades. Reach behind you with your left hand and try to touch your fingertips together behind your back. If they don't touch, have a partner eyeball how many inches apart they are. Repeat this test with your left hand overhead and your right hand reaching around.

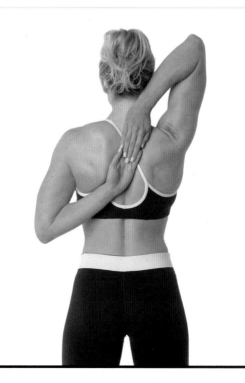

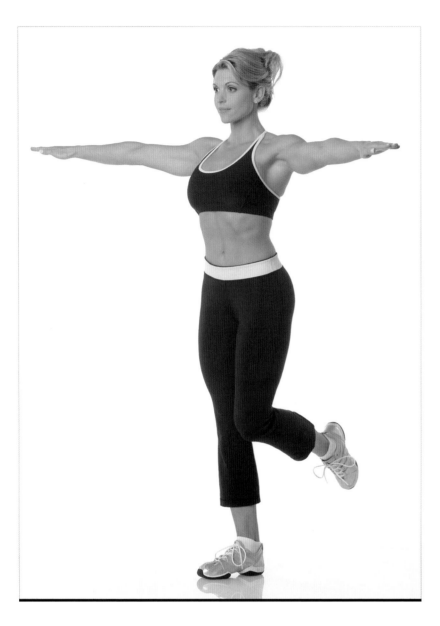

Extra Credit: Balance Test

Tests: Balance and stability

Instructions: Do this test on both sides.

Stand with your knees slightly bent, arms at your sides. Pick one foot up off the floor, lifting your heel behind you, and balance on one leg for as long as you can. Have a partner time you. If this is easy for you, bring your arms straight out to the sides at shoulder height (as shown). If this is still easy for you, place both hands behind your head, elbows bent.

YOUR WEIGHT

It's a good idea to know your starting point when it comes to scale weight. So using a standard bathroom scale, record your weight today. Mark it down in your workout journal underneath your measurements, and then *put the scale away*! I am not a big advocate of weighing yourself all the time. People get so hung up on their scale weight, but really, it's a highly inaccurate measure of progress. As you'll learn in later chapters, muscle weighs significantly more than fat, and while your scale weight might stay the same, your body fat may be melting away. A better way to gauge progress is by checking how your clothes fit. If a pair of size 10 pants is tight one week, see how it fits the next week, and the next, and the next. Clothing is a much more accurate measure of fat loss and body composition changes than a scale.

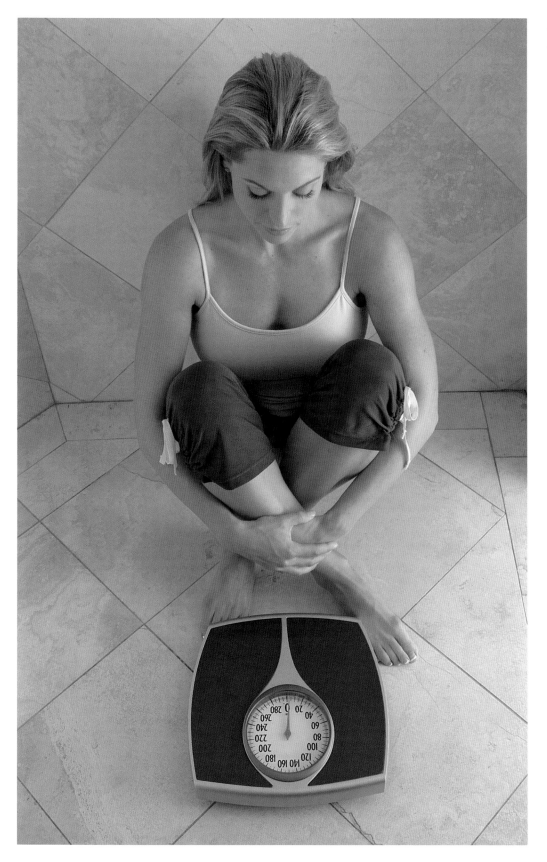

I weighed myself this morning and I was 143, but this afternoon I was 148! How can I gain 5 pounds in only 6 hours? This is why I don't want people weighing themselves too often! Talk about discouraging. Of course you didn't gain 5 pounds of fat in 6 hours. That is physically impossible. But your scale weight can fluctuate up to 5 pounds in a 24-hour period, depending on what you eat, how much you drink, whether it's "that time of the month," whether you've gone to the bathroom yet, or whether you're stressed out. All these things can add to your total scale weight, which measures how hard gravity is pulling your total body mass (water, food, fat, muscle, organs, and bones) toward the center of the earth. A scale does not tell you if you're losing body fat or if you're bloated. It only tells you how heavy you are right now. This is why I discourage daily weighing—it's disheartening and depressing!

Here is a sure-fire way to make peace with your scale and get over it once and for all! For one week only, you're allowed to obsess about weighing yourself. Once you're done with this week, though, you have to get over it and put that scale away! Promise? OK. Now, weigh yourself several times a day for an entire week, and write down your results on a piece of paper or in your journal. Noting your daily fluctuations will make you realize how inconsistent and inaccurate the scale really is. I did a little three-day test myself. Check out my results, below.

Obviously I didn't gain or lose 4 pounds of body fat in three days! My scale weight fluctuated according to how much water I was retaining or expelling, what I ate, and what time of day it was. Try this experiment for yourself, make peace with your scale, then put the darn thing away!

When I weighed myself		My weight
Monday	First thing in morning	121 pounds
	10 minutes later (after peeing!)	120 pounds
	Early afternoon (after drinking tons of water)	121 pounds
	Before bed (had Chinese food for dinner)	122 pounds
Tuesday	First thing in the morning	123 pounds
	Afternoon (after drinking tons of water)	122 pounds
	Before bed (had asparagus for dinner)	124 pounds
Wednesday	First thing in the morning	121 pounds
	10 minutes later (after peeing)	120 pounds

SUMMARY

You should know your starting point when beginning a fitness program, whether you're a former athlete or a new recruit to healthy living. Though it may be daunting, taking your measurements, weighing yourself, and performing the fitness tests will give you a good idea of both your limitations and your capabilities! Your initial numbers may be embarrassing or depressing, but don't dwell on the negative—instead look to the future and be inspired. You've got nowhere to go from here but up!

HOMEWORK

1. Spend some time looking at the numbers you wrote down for your initial fitness tests, measurements, and weight. How do these numbers make you feel? Write down your thoughts about these numbers and measurements, including anything negative or positive you're feeling about yourself and your results.
2. Once you've gotten out all your negative feelings, write an intention for change. What do you plan to do about these numbers? How will you change them for the better in the next twelve weeks? Be as specific as possible to help set some realistic and achievable goals.
3. Take the scale test I described in the Burning Question section on page 42. Record your results in your journal and keep them to remind you that the scale is very inaccurate!
4. Today and for the next week, have a protein with every meal. Protein helps build muscle and keeps you fuller longer during the day. For more information on protein and its role in the body, turn to page 190!

Extra Credit

Have a friend take a Polaroid picture of you from the front, side, and back. These are your official "before" pictures. Write down ten words you'd use to describe the person in these pictures in your journal. Stash these photos and paper away for now—you'll revisit them again in twelve weeks.

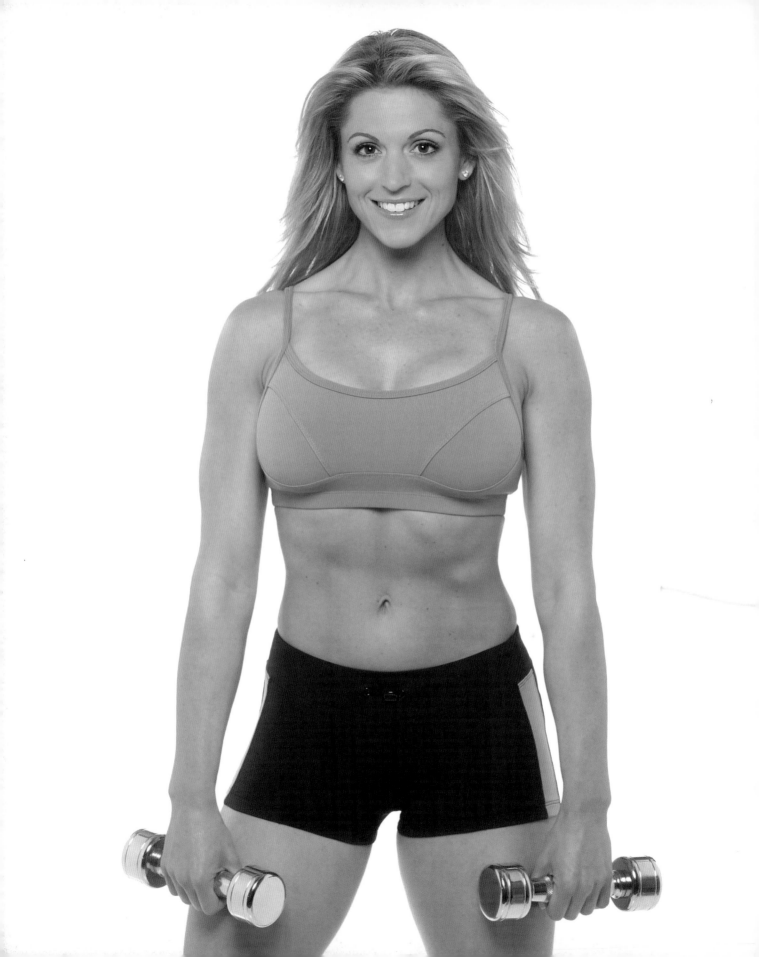

Your Workout

WELCOME TO YOUR WORKOUTS! This section is dedicated to answering all your questions about exercise, including: How often should you work out? What should you do? How do you start? Fitness is a marathon, not a sprint, and *Your Body, Your Life* offers a progressive system of slow and steady weight loss, instrumental in creating lasting physical changes. The workout plans are divided into three levels, each building on the last as you improve and become more fit. You'll advance gradually, building strength and endurance while simultaneously toning and slimming your body. No matter what your abilities, you'll find a challenging workout to suit your needs!

CHAPTER **7**

Understand It

Fun Fact

Muscle cells burn calories just by *being*!

The Miracle of Music

I don't know about you, but I can't exercise without music! Music sets the mood for my workouts, jazzing me up to do cardio or lift weights, or mellowing me out to stretch and work on my flexibility. I have different playlists on my iPod that I change all the time to suit my mood and activity. Check out some of my tune lists on my Web site, www.kimlyons.com!

Most women believe the way to lose weight is to do cardio, cardio, and more cardio. This was the case with Maria. She set off on her quest to lose weight without much erudition or pointed direction, and did tons of cardio. Six days a week she walked, jogged, and rode the stationary bike for 45–60 minutes at a time. At first, she lost a bunch of weight; excited, she did more cardio. But after a few months, she stopped losing weight and her progress plateaued. In addition, her hips and knees were sore and achy, and she was bored stiff with her routine. Confused and discouraged, Maria came to me for advice. I suggested cutting her cardio down to twice a week and adding resistance and flexibility training to her program three days a week. She was dubious about this plan, since she hadn't lifted weights before and was afraid of "getting big." But since her current program wasn't working, she figured she'd give mine a try.

In the next several weeks, Maria's body began to change. Her legs slimmed down, her waist got smaller, and her arms gained shape and definition. Although she had not lost any weight on the scale, she was fitting into clothes several sizes smaller, which was amazing, she said, because she was also eating a lot more food. Moreover, her hip and knee pain had all but disappeared. She was excited about these transformations but was still confused as to how they happened. Why did her cardio stop working? How could she weigh the same but be smaller? How could she eat so much food without gaining weight? We sat down and discussed her questions.

In Maria's original program, she was doing only cardio. This worked at first because her body was not yet used to this stimulus and responded by dropping weight. But soon, her body adapted to this routine, and her endless hours of cardio were for nothing. In fitness, three elements need to be in balance: cardiovascular work, resistance training, and flexibility training. Think of these elements as legs on a triangle. If one of them is neglected or overdone, the triangle is lopsided and unbalanced. The same goes for your fitness program: Each element has to be in balance to create a fit, healthy body. Because Maria was doing only cardio, her triangle was way out of balance.

What Maria didn't realize is that cardio is not the only element of fitness that burns calories: Resistance training also burns tons of calories, especially during the "afterburn" that occurs in the days following your workout. Your body takes one to two days to "recover" from a resistance workout, expending tons of energy (i.e., calories!) on repairing and rebuilding tissues, and trying to return to a "resting state," the state it was in before a workout. Resistance training also changes your body composition, adding more muscle cells and increasing your metabolic rate. This is why Maria was able to eat more food—her calories were going to build and maintain her new muscle tissue and were being used up as fuel instead of being stored. And since Maria's new muscle was more dense than fat, her scale weight didn't change, but she got smaller and tighter and fit into pants she hadn't worn in years. She also stretched after every workout, releasing her tight muscles and eliminating her joint pain.

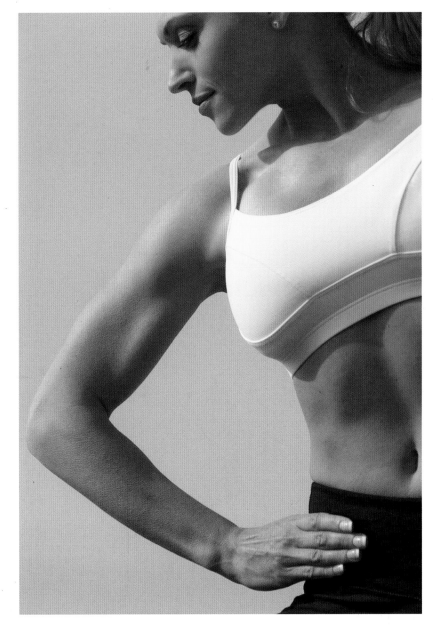

Resistance training gives you the toned muscles you always wanted!

BENEFITS OF . . .

LIFTING WEIGHTS

- increased muscle strength, power, and endurance
- increased bone density
- increased strength of tendons and ligaments
- decreased blood pressure, resting heart rate, and body fat
- improved balance, posture, and coordination
- elevated metabolism
- improved self-esteem
- reduced risk of injury

End Result: A tight, hot body!

CARDIOVASCULAR TRAINING

- increased endurance, blood flow, and skeletal strength
- decreased body fat and blood pressure
- improved heart function
- decreased anxiety, depression, and tension
- lowered risk of cardiovascular disease, obesity, hypertension, and high cholesterol

End Result: A tighter body, and smaller clothing sizes!

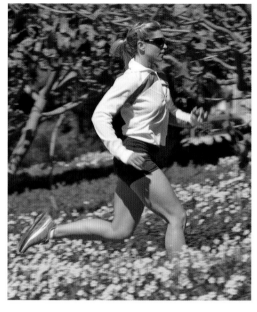

Cardio burns away body fat!

know it or not, it's this muscle tissue that gives you the washboard abs or toned arms you dream about!

Fun Fact

Women especially benefit from weight training because it increases bone density and strength, preventing and sometimes even reversing osteoporosis!

Now Maria tells everyone about how balanced fitness changed her physique. The combination of resistance training, cardiovascular work, and stretching worked wonders for her and enabled her to fit into size 8 pants in six months!

THE FITNESS TRIANGLE

The *Your Body, Your Life* program includes all three elements of fitness. Let's check each one out individually.

Resistance Training

Resistance training is important on so many levels. It improves strength, coordination, and balance, reduces the risk of many diseases, and adds quality lean muscle tissue to your frame. Whether you

BURNING QUESTION

Do I have to lift weights? I want to be toned, but I'm afraid of getting big. So you want to be "toned." What does that mean? Well, you can't tone fat. Fat just sits there looking fat! But you can tone muscle. And how do you tone muscle? By lifting weights. So yes, in order to get toned, you have to lift weights. But don't be scared of pumping a little iron: Resistance training will not make a woman look like a man. Women simply don't have the hormonal constitution to get bodybuilder big. Instead, your muscles will become more shapely, giving you the "tone" you're talking about. And since a pound of muscle takes up less space than a pound of fat, your dress size will shrink. Moreover, everyday tasks will become easier as you become stronger, and your body will look and feel more youthful!

Cardiovascular Training

Cardiovascular training (or cardio for short) is just that—training your heart, lungs, and circulatory system to work better and more efficiently. Cardio reduces stress and anxiety, decreases blood pressure, and most of all burns calories! If you're lifting weights regularly, you'll still need to do cardio to strip away the body fat from on top of those muscles to show them off!

Does a pound of muscle weigh more than a pound of fat? No! It's a trick question. A pound is a pound, whether it's a pound of feathers or a pound of chicken. The difference is the amount of space that a pound takes up: A pound of chicken fits neatly in a baking dish, whereas a pound of feathers might fill your bathroom. On your body, a pound of muscle is very dense, so it takes up less space than a pound of body fat. If you have 5 pounds of muscle on your frame, you will appear smaller and tighter than you would if you had 5 pounds of fat in the same place.

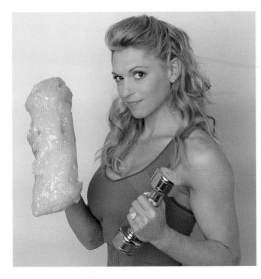

Look at the difference in size between a 5-pound weight and a scale model of 5 pounds of body fat!

Flexibility

Flexibility is probably the most overlooked aspect of fitness, but while it's less glamorous than cardio and strength training, it is no less important. Flexibility is defined as a joint's ability to move through its full range of motion. This means being able to bend, flex, and move comfortably in all directions, allowing you to work out harder and more efficiently, ultimately burning more calories!

BENEFITS OF . . .

FLEXIBILITY TRAINING
- increased range of motion
- decreased risk of injury
- reduced muscle soreness and back pain
- improved muscle balance, posture, and physical performance
- increased circulation and relaxation

End Result: Better workouts and improved quality of life!

CIRCUIT TRAINING
- saves time
- incorporates cardio and resistance training in one workout
- burns tons of calories
- works your heart, lungs, and muscles all at once
engages your mind as well as your muscles

End Result: An effective, time-efficient, calorie-blasting way to train!

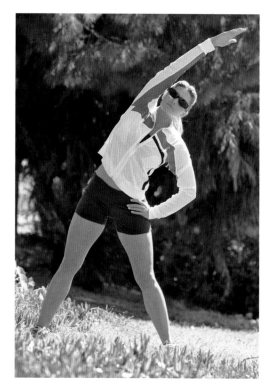

Stretch after exercise for the best results!

Fun Fact

Recent research suggests that to get maximum power from your muscles, you should stretch after you work out, and not before!

BURNING QUESTION

What are yoga, tai chi, and Pilates? Yoga is a practice that originated in India thousands of years ago that combines physical postures with breathing and meditation to relax, stretch, and strengthen the body and mind. Tai chi resembles a moving, meditative form of yoga, consisting of moves derived from martial arts performed in a slow and graceful way. Like yoga, tai chi serves to relax and align the body. Pilates, which is used to strengthen the body's core, looks like a cross between yoga and standard flexibility training and involves mat exercises, machine-assisted exercises, or both. Any of these practices is great for participants of all levels who want to stretch, strengthen, and unwind.

CIRCUIT TRAINING

At this point you've got a pretty good grasp of the three elements needed to create a fit and healthy body. Now let's put them all together into one simple system: circuit training.

Circuit training is an effective, efficient way to work out. The *Your Body, Your Life* workout circuits alternate between lower-body resistance-training moves (to elevate your heart rate) and upper-body moves (to allow you to recover), giving you an interval training effect that burns tons of calories and develops incredible endurance! Because of the continuous nature of circuit training, you'll get all the benefits of resistance training, have a great cardiovascular workout, and maximize your training time. After your workout circuit, you'll perform a flexibility circuit, which stretches all your major muscle groups, improving range of motion, decreasing muscle soreness, and helping alleviate chronic pain.

SUMMARY

To keep your fitness triangle in balance and get the best results possible from the *Your Body, Your Life* program, you need to incorporate resistance training, cardiovascular activity, and flexibility work into your schedule. Resistance training will build lean muscle mass, cardio will strip away body fat, and flexibility will keep your new body supple and injury free. All three elements can be combined in circuits that build endurance, burn calories, and save time!

HOMEWORK

1. Take a few moments to think back on your previous workout programs. Did they include all three elements of fitness? Write out what might have been missing, and be sure to include those elements in your plan this go-round.
2. The next time you're feeling crabby or sad, do some cardio! Notice whether your mood changes for the better.
3. Today and the rest of this week, try to eat a meal or snack every 3–4 hours. To read more about the importance of meal timing, turn to page 208!

Extra Credit

Make yourself three music playlists for your MP3 player or iPod: one for resistance training, one for cardio, and one for stretching. Use music you like that gets you excited and motivated to work out.

CLIENT CORNER

KISS MY KNEECAPS, BY CODY

In college I played baseball and swam the 100 meters, and was so flexible that I could fold in half and kiss my kneecaps while sitting on the floor. That impressed the girls! But after graduation, life caught up with me. I took a desk job and worked out sporadically at best. I slowly got more and more out of shape, and my back was sore and tight from sitting all the time. By the time I started training with Kim, I was as stiff as a board. I could barely reach around to get into the sleeves of my sport coat, and touching my toes? Forget it!

Kim made it her mission to help me regain some of my collegiate flexibility. I am not a yoga dude, so she showed me some simple stretches to do after my workouts or even at work if I had been sitting for a while and was feeling tight. And whaddya know—in a month I was able to touch my shins, and the month after that I reached my shoelaces! Miraculous. Not only that, but my back pain began to abate, and these days it is nearly gone. I am able to work out better now that my flexibility has improved. I have a greater range of motion through my hips and hamstrings, making moves such as squats more effective and getting me to my goals more quickly. My next goal: to once again kiss my kneecaps, and hopefully impress some girls!

AN ODE TO CIRCUITS, BY MY CLIENTS

Kim's circuit training is my absolute favorite! I get bored really easily and am not a gym rat at all. I hate getting on the cardio machines where you're on there for an hour—it's really boring. So when Kim showed me that I can do twenty different exercises, hit all my body parts, lose weight, and burn a ton of calories without sitting on the treadmill for an hour, I said, "Where do I sign up?" —Pam

Anyone can do Kim's circuits and get a great workout. You can do them when you're 300 pounds and work up a good sweat, and you can do them when you're 200 pounds and work up a good sweat by simply changing the intensity. You can do them in your hotel room, in your house, or at the gym, they're so versatile. —Jaron

Before Kim, I had never done anything like circuit training, and I have to be honest—at first I hated the hell out of squats and lunges! They were so hard for me, and I dreaded doing them. But once I began to see results, I loved the circuits, and these days, squats and lunges are my favorites! They do so much to change your physique that I never go a week without doing them. —Kai

CHAPTER 8

Plan It

As you learned in Chapter 7, the *Your Body, Your Life* workout program uses circuit training as the basis for all workouts. Here's how your workouts are going to play out, no matter what your starting level.

THE PLAN

There are three levels in the *Your Body, Your Life* workout program:

• **Level I** uses the basics—single-joint moves to develop a solid base of strength and endurance.
• **Level II** takes it up a notch, combining two or more Level I moves into "double moves," increasing the difficulty and calorie burn of the workout.
• **Level III** takes it one step farther, adding an element of balance or core strength to Level I and II moves for a calorie-scorching, total-body workout you'll love!

The moves for all three workout levels are arranged into circuits. In each circuit,

you'll progress from one exercise to the next with minimal rest between sets, giving you all the benefits of resistance training while simultaneously giving you a great cardio workout.

Within each level you'll find four separate workouts:

• **Two Total-Body Circuit Workouts,** to work all the muscles of the body
• **One Lower-Body/Cardio Workout,** to focus on the legs, core, and cardiovascular system
• **One Trouble Spots Workout,** for zoning in on the hips, glutes, abs, and thighs

Do each of these workouts at least once during a given week for maximum results.

SCHEDULE

On the next two pages, you'll find a suggested twelve-week schedule for the *Your Body, Your Life* workout program. This schedule is only suggested because there are no rules about how long you stay at each

Level I

WEEK	MONDAY	TUESDAY	WEDNESDAY	THURSDAY	FRIDAY	SATURDAY	SUNDAY
1	Circuit 1	Trouble Spots	Rest	Circuit 2	Rest	Lower Body/Cardio	Rest
2	Circuit 1	Trouble Spots	Rest	Circuit 2	Rest	Lower Body/Cardio	Rest
3	Circuit 1	Trouble Spots	Rest	Circuit 2	Optional Cardio	Lower Body/Cardio	Rest
4	Circuit 1	Trouble Spots	Rest	Circuit 2	Optional Cardio	Lower Body/Cardio	Rest

Level II

WEEK	MONDAY	TUESDAY	WEDNESDAY	THURSDAY	FRIDAY	SATURDAY	SUNDAY
1	Circuit 1and Trouble Spots	Lower Body/ Cardio	Rest	Circuit 2	Cardio	Rest or Lower Body/Cardio	Rest
2	Circuit 1and Trouble Spots	Lower Body/ Cardio	Rest	Circuit 2	Cardio	Rest or Lower Body/Cardio	Rest
3	Circuit 1	Lower Body/ Cardio	Rest	Circuit 2 and Trouble Spots	Cardio	Rest or Lower Body/Cardio	Rest
4	Circuit 1	Lower Body/ Cardio	Rest	Circuit 2 and Trouble Spots	Cardio	Rest or Lower Body/Cardio	Rest

Level III

WEEK	MONDAY	TUESDAY	WEDNESDAY	THURSDAY	FRIDAY	SATURDAY	SUNDAY
1	Circuit 1	Lower Body/ Cardio	Circuit 2 and Cardio	Rest	Lower Body/ Cardio and Trouble Spots	Either Circuit 1 or Circuit 2	Rest
2	Circuit 1	Lower Body/ Cardio	Circuit 2 and Cardio	Rest	Lower Body/ Cardio and Trouble Spots	Either Circuit 1 or Circuit 2	Rest
3	Circuit 1 and Trouble Spots	Lower Body/ Cardio	Circuit 2 and Cardio	Rest	Lower Body/ Cardio and Trouble Spots	Either Circuit 1 or Circuit 2	Rest
4	Circuit 1 and Trouble Spots	Lower Body/ Cardio	Circuit 2 and Cardio	Rest	Lower Body/ Cardio and Trouble Spots	Either Circuit 1 or Circuit 2	Rest

level. If you spend all twelve weeks at Level I, so be it! If you speed through Level I in two weeks, great! If you start Level III, get overwhelmed, and go back to Level II, fabulous! The point is not to chain you to an unyielding workout schedule; it's to help you establish a habit of regular exercise by doing three to five workouts every week.

Even so, I encourage everyone to start at Level I. The moves you'll learn in this section will be incorporated in Levels II and III, and it's a good idea to familiarize yourself with them for one or two weeks before moving up a notch.

A Note on Cardio

You'll notice "Cardio" marked in your schedule once a week. During this time, do an activity that elevates your heart rate and keeps it there for the whole workout. The purpose here is to burn a few more calories while giving your heart and lungs

a different kind of stimulus than the circuits do, increasing your fitness level.

A Note on Rest Days

The only part of the schedule to which I insist you adhere are your Rest Days. You must take at least two days a week completely off from working out to rebuild and repair your muscles and tissues, and avoid overuse injuries and overtraining. On Rest Days, you can do something mildly active such as 30 minutes of flexibility training, or playing outside with your kids, but don't schedule hard workouts if your body is telling you it needs time off.

BURNING QUESTION
I work out every day for 2 hours and have stopped losing weight! What happened?
You're overtraining. While it might seem like a good idea to work out more and for

a longer period of time to accelerate weight loss, your body can handle only so much breakdown. Think of a car: Your oil light comes on one day. Instead of taking it to the shop and getting it fixed, you ignore it. The next day, your oil pan is dry and smoke starts coming out of the hood. You again choose to ignore it. The third day, the engine seizes up and the car stops moving. This is similar to what happens in your body if you ignore the signs of overtraining (listed below). If you don't give your body the rest it needs, it will stop making progress and may even break down to the point of chronic or severe injury. Instead of getting to that point, take at least two full days off from training every week and work out no more than 60 minutes per session.

Signs of Overtraining
• lack of visible progress
• diminished endurance, strength, or speed
• increased irritability and moodiness
• insomnia
• chronic nagging aches and pains
• lack of energy and loss of enthusiasm
• decreased appetite
• headaches

A Note on Flexibility
In my perfect world, you'd do 30 minutes of flexibility training every day! But in reality, I will settle for 10–15 dedicated minutes of stretching after every workout. Stretching will increase flexibility, decrease muscle soreness, and improve recovery. Stretch the muscles used during the workout, and those that are exceptionally sore or tight from previous workouts. You'll find a number of flexibility moves in Chapter 9 as well as a sample total-body stretching circuit.

A Note on Intensity
Your workouts will be only as hard as you make them. Remember: The more intense a workout, the more calories you will burn, so give each and every workout your all. To measure your intensity, I recommend using the rate of perceived exertion (RPE) scale (see page 56). This scale measures how hard you feel you're working based on physical sensations such as heart rate, breathing rate, sweat rate, and muscle fatigue. Although this is a subjective scale, it's usually pretty accurate.

Your Cardio and Trouble Spots workouts should fall between a 3 and a 5 on this scale, and your circuit workouts between a 6 and an 8. Some of you might find that your Lower-Body/Cardio workouts hover around 9; this is fine. But make sure you give yourself enough time between sets to recover to around a level 6.

Suggested Cardio Activities

Indoors	Outdoors
Walking, jogging, running on a treadmill	Walking, jogging, running outside
Rowing machine	Kayaking
Elliptical trainer	In-line skating
Swimming	Surfing
Stairmaster	Stair or hill walking/running
Stationary bike	Road/mountain biking
Cross-country ski machine	Cross-country skiing

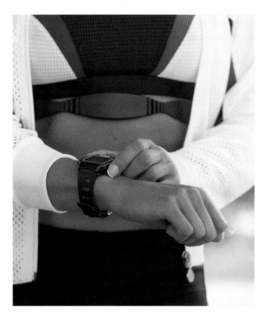

RPE Scale

Level	Effort level
0	Nothing at all
1–2	Very easy; you can converse with no effort
3	Easy; you can converse with almost no effort
4	Moderately easy; you can converse with little effort
5	Moderate; conversation requires some effort
6	Moderately hard; conversation requires quite a bit of effort
7	Difficult; conversation requires quite a lot of effort
8	Very difficult; conversation requires maximum effort
9–10	Peak effort; no-talking zone

BURNING QUESTION

What are heart rate monitors? Heart rate monitors consist of two pieces—an adjustable chest band and a wristwatch—that continually monitor and display your current working heart rate. More intricate monitors also calculate calories burned during a workout, or even during the course of an entire day! They do cost a bit of money and require some setting up, but they are a great way to measure exact workout intensity and ensure steady progress. I never do a workout without mine! It keeps me on track with my goals and reminds me if I am not training hard enough.

RULES AND REGS

For all your workouts, follow these rules and regs for the safest, most effective session possible:

Rules for Circuit Training

Always warm up for 5–10 minutes with some light cardio such as walking, jogging, or riding a stationary bike before doing your circuits. This moves blood and heat into your muscles and joints, properly preparing the body for work.

Avoid the use of momentum when lifting weights. Move through each repetition of an exercise slowly and deliberately, maintaining an even pace.

Use proper form for all exercises. If you're not sure of the form for a move, reread the description given, and do the move in front of a mirror. Make sure your body position looks similar to the one shown in the photograph.

Use a full range of motion for each exercise. Don't stop short on any move, or "cheat" a repetition by using other muscles to do the lift. Use a complete range of motion as depicted in the workout photographs for the best results.

Always cool down for 5–10 minutes after exercising. This allows the blood to return to other parts of the body, letting your body return to a resting state.

Stretch after you lift for at least 10–15 minutes, more if possible, to reduce next-day soreness and increase flexibility. Always stretch *after* exercise, when your muscles are warm and supple. Focus on the muscles used during the workout, as well as any others that are sore or stiff from previous workouts.

Rules for Cardio

Warm up and cool down for 5–10 minutes around your cardio session. The warm-up gets blood and heat into the muscles and prepares the body for exercise, and the cool-down allows your heart rate to return to normal and your body to return to a resting state.

Stretch for 5–10 minutes after your workout. Focus on the large muscles of the body such as the legs, back, shoulders, and core.

Change your routine often. Your body (and brain!) will get bored quickly if you always do the same thing. Do different kinds of cardio each week to use different muscles and keep progressing.

Do something you like! This is so important—if you don't like the activity you're doing, you're less likely to do it. If you hate running, don't run! Go swimming, take an aerobics class, or hike in the mountains instead.

A LITTLE MATH

If you like an extra challenge, figure out your target heart rate (THR) zone. This zone represents the rate at which your heart should be beating (beats per minutes—BPM) in order to more efficiently lose weight. First, find your maximum heart rate using this formula:

220 − Your Age = Maximum Heart Rate (MHR)

Then figure out your THR by multiplying a percentage of effort by your MHR. Cardio should be done at 65 percent to 80 percent of your MHR; circuit workouts should be between 60 percent and 90 percent of your MHR.

Cardio Zone: (MHR × 65%) to (MHR × 80%) = THR

Circuit Zone: (MHR × 60%) to (MHR × 90%) = THR

Example—Betsy, a Thirty-Year-Old Woman: 220 − 30 = 190 MHR

Cardio Zone: (190 × .65) to (190 × .80) = 123.5 to 152 = THR

Circuit Zone: (190 × .60) to (190 × .90) = 114 to 171 = THR

Betsy's maximum heart rate is 190 beats per minute. Her target heart rate should be between 123 and 152 beats per minute during cardio and between 114 and 171 for circuits.

Rules for Stretching

Warm up before stretching. Muscles are like taffy: Try to stretch them when they are cold, and they'll snap! Stretch them when they are warm, and they'll elongate easily. Reserve your flexibility work for after your exercise session, or do 5–10 minutes of light cardio beforehand.

Stretch to the limit of your range of motion, not to the point of pain. You don't have to become Gumby; just work to increase your own personal range of motion. Stretch and hold at the point of resistance, slowly increasing your stretch as you breathe.

Hold each stretch for 15–30 seconds. Research indicates that you'll gain the most benefit by holding a position for at least this long.

Breathe deeply. Consciously inhale and exhale while holding each stretch. This will help deliver oxygen to the stretching muscles while helping you relax.

Avoid bouncing (ballistic stretching). This harsh technique can cause trauma to muscle cells, ligaments, and tendons, tempting injury.

SUMMARY

Circuit training is a great way to work out! It combines the strengthening elements of resistance training with the fat-burning elements of cardio activity and packages them into a time-efficient, fun workout! Follow the guidelines and rules in this chapter, and you'll always have a great, safe workout!

HOMEWORK

1. Look over the suggested workout schedules listed on pages 53 and 54. Decide which one might be most appropriate for you. The take out your workout journal and pencil in your workouts for your first week right now!
2. If you're feeling energetic, go out and do your cardio workout today, right now, and I mean immediately! Afterward, write down how it went in your workout journal.
3. Today and for the rest of this week, try to cut out as much sugar and excess sodium from your diet as possible. To read more about the effects of sugar and sodium on the body, turn to pages 199 and 203!

Extra Credit

Buy a heart rate monitor to use for your workouts. Then, using the formula on page 57, determine your target heart rate range. Wear your monitor each time you work out, and write down in your workout journal how successful you were at staying in your range.

CHAPTER 9

Work It

LEVEL I

Welcome to your beginning workouts! In Level I you'll be learning the basics. All the moves here are "single moves," meaning you're exercising only one body part at a time—biceps, shoulders, legs, abs, and so on. You'll see these moves again in Levels II and III, so learn them well!

Level I Instructions

Points of Focus
- warming up and cooling down properly
- using proper form
- learning movement patterns for basic exercises
- breathing while lifting
- using full range of motion
- performing slow, controlled repetitions

Who Is This Level For?

Everyone! Absolute beginners and previous exercisers alike should begin here and learn these moves thoroughly. You might feel awkward at first as you try new things, but in a few weeks, these moves will become second nature!

Circuit Works

1. Try to do each move for 30 seconds. This is going to be hard for many of you, so don't feel badly if you have to take breaks at first. Make it your future goal to do a full 30 seconds without stopping. Once you've accomplished that goal, pick up the next heaviest set of dumbbells and start again!

2. In between moves, take a 60-second rest. During this time, walk around, sip some water, or stretch a little, but don't sit down! You want to keep your heart rate elevated so you burn more calories. *Note:* You may need a little more time to recover when doing the Lower Body/Cardio workouts, which can elevate your heart rate quickly. Pace yourself and take breaks when needed.

3. During the first few weeks, go through each circuit once. As you get stronger and your coordination improves, go through each circuit twice. By the end of the month, you should be able to do each routine two to three times!

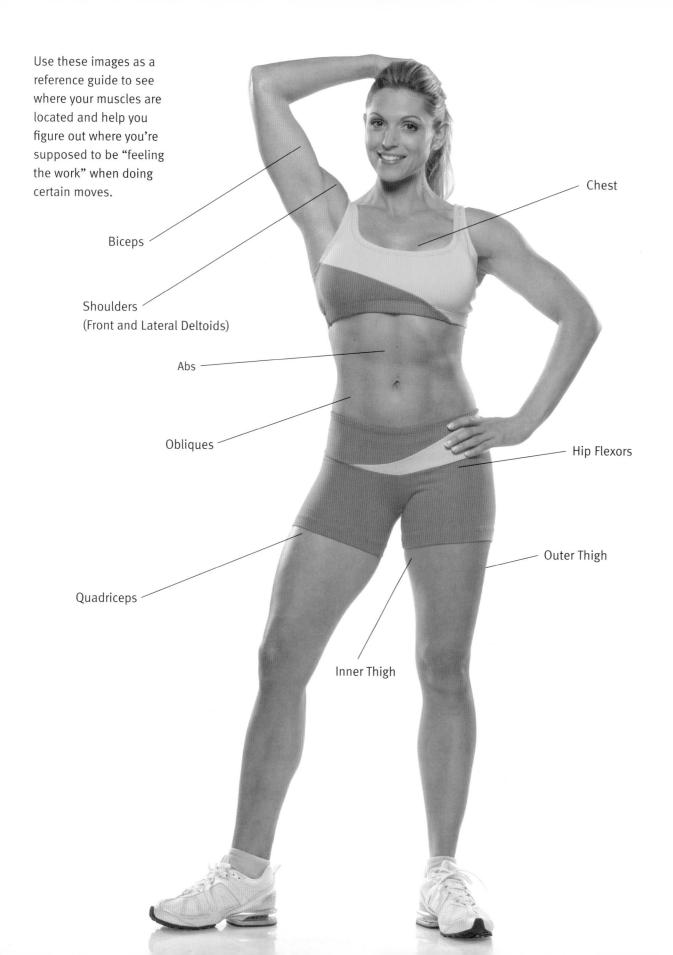

Use these images as a reference guide to see where your muscles are located and help you figure out where you're supposed to be "feeling the work" when doing certain moves.

Chest

Biceps

Shoulders
(Front and Lateral Deltoids)

Abs

Obliques

Hip Flexors

Outer Thigh

Quadriceps

Inner Thigh

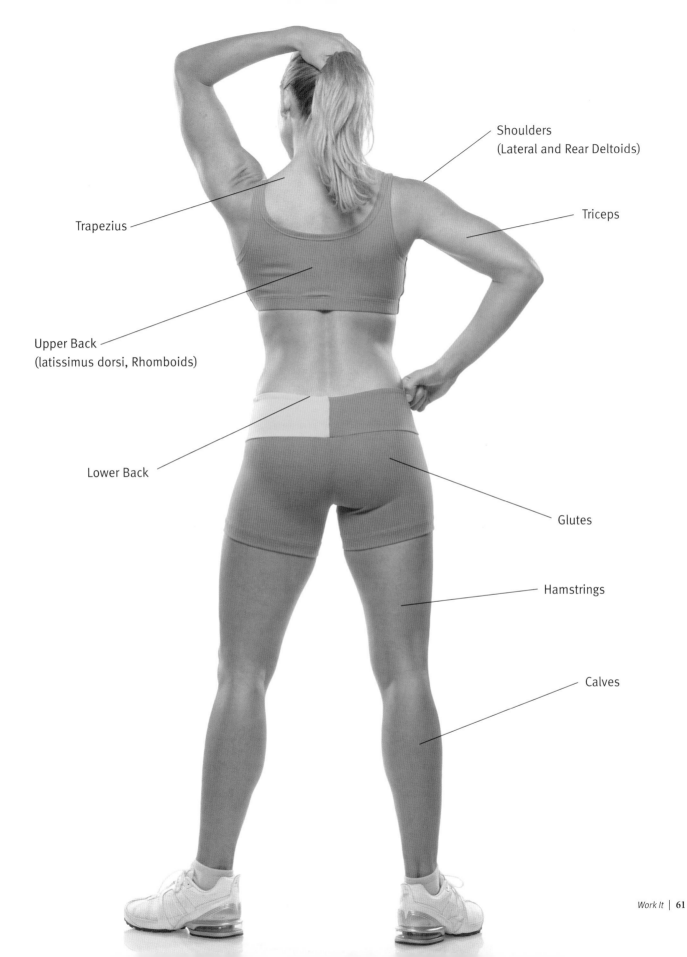

Shoulders
(Lateral and Rear Deltoids)

Triceps

Trapezius

Upper Back
(latissimus dorsi, Rhomboids)

Lower Back

Glutes

Hamstrings

Calves

Circuit Math

    10 moves @ 30 seconds each
+ 60 seconds rest in between moves
= 15 minutes each circuit (once through)

Which Weights?

Start with your smallest set of weights (between 3 and 5 pounds), and go up or down from there, according to how you feel. Once you can complete 30 full seconds without stopping with a particular set of weights, it's time to move up.

Note: Absolute beginners can do the first week without weights to get used to the movement patterns and learn correct form.

Cardio Rx

Do at least 20 continuous minutes of cardio for your workouts this month.

Good Level I Cardio Ideas
• walking
• elliptical trainer with no arms
• biking
• in-line skating
• swimming

Note: Remember to do 5–10 minutes of warm-up and cool-down in addition to the 20 minutes of cardio work!

Biceps Curl

Muscles worked: Biceps

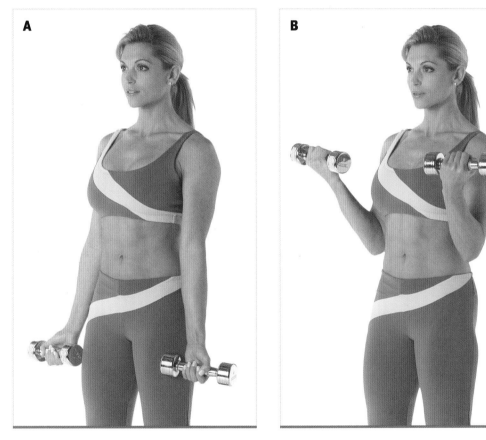

Beginner's Tip
Don't use your back to do this lift. Focus on isolating your biceps muscles to curl the weights.

A. Stand with your feet hip-width apart and your knees slightly bent, and hold a pair of dumbbells in front of your thighs, palms facing up.

B. Slowly curl the weights up toward your shoulders, keeping your elbows in tight to your body. Resist the pull of gravity as you lower the dumbbells back to the start.

Strongman Curl

Muscles worked: Biceps, shoulders (lateral deltoids)

Beginner's Tip
Don't let your elbows drop below shoulder level. Keep them raised and strong throughout the move.

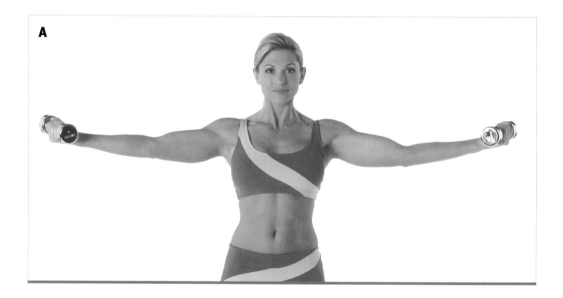

A. Stand with your feet hip-width apart, knees slightly bent. Hold a pair of dumb-bells at shoulder height, arms held straight out and parallel to the floor, palms facing the ceiling.

B. Keep your upper arms steady as you slowly curl the dumbbells in toward your head. Reverse the motion to return to the start.

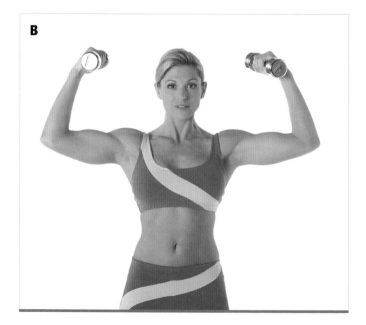

Overhead Triceps Extension

Muscles worked: Triceps

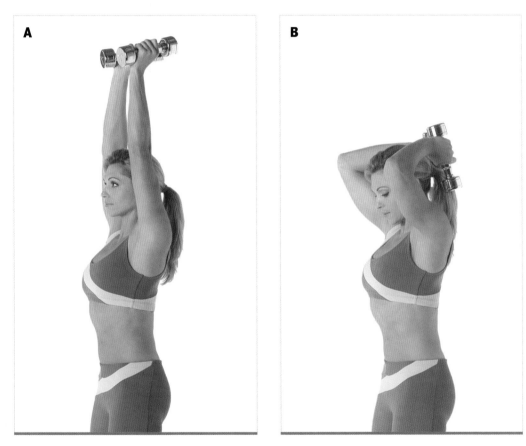

Beginner's Tip
Control your weights! It hurts like heck if you allow them to drop freely and bang you in the noggin! I like to dip my chin toward my chest slightly to make room back there for the weights.

A. Stand with your feet hip-width apart and your knees slightly bent, and hold a pair of dumbbells overhead, arms straight, elbows close to your ears.

B. Slowly bend your elbows, dropping the weights behind your head, then extend your arms overhead to return to the start position.

Upright Row

Muscles worked: Shoulders, trapezius

Beginner's Tip
Even though you're pulling the weights up toward your chin, try not to shrug your shoulders. Keep your neck and shoulders relaxed and neutral throughout the move.

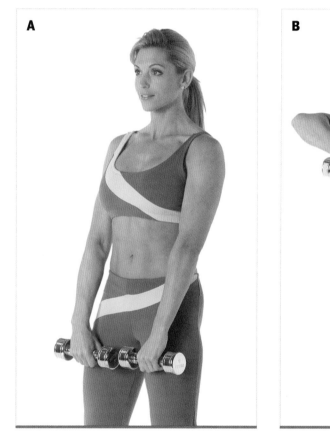

A. Stand with your feet hip-width apart and your knees slightly bent, and hold a pair of dumbbells close together in front of you, palms facing your thighs.

B. Lift the dumbbells up toward your chin, leading the motion with your elbows and keeping your shoulders down and back. When the weights reach your clavicles, slowly reverse the motion to come back to the start.

Overhead Shoulder Press

Muscles worked: Shoulders (front and lateral deltoids)

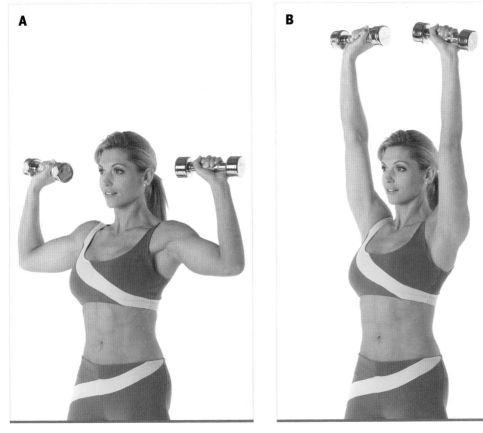

Beginner's Tip
It's tricky to learn how to push things over your head, so watch yourself in a mirror here to make sure the weights are moving up and down in a straight line.

A. Stand with your feet hip-width apart and your knees slightly bent, and hold a pair of dumbbells at ear level, elbows down, wrists stacked over elbows, and palms facing forward.

B. Straighten your arms and press the weights up overhead until your arms reach full extension. Slowly reverse the motion to lower the weights back to the start.

Lateral Shoulder Raise

Muscles worked: Shoulders (lateral deltoids)

Beginner's Tip

If you seesaw during this move, you're using your back to pull the weights up. Keep your core strong and your back steady, and lift only with your shoulders.

A. Stand with your feet hip-width apart and your knees slightly bent, and hold a pair of dumbbells in front of your thighs. Bend your elbows slightly and turn your palms to face each other.

B. Lift the weights up and out to the sides, leading the motion with your elbows. Raise the weights to shoulder height, then slowly lower them to the start, resisting the pull of gravity on the return.

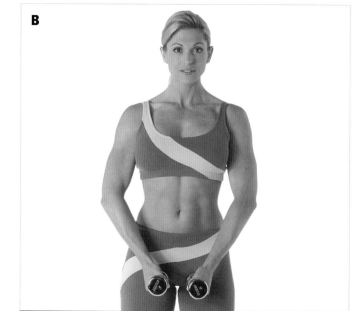

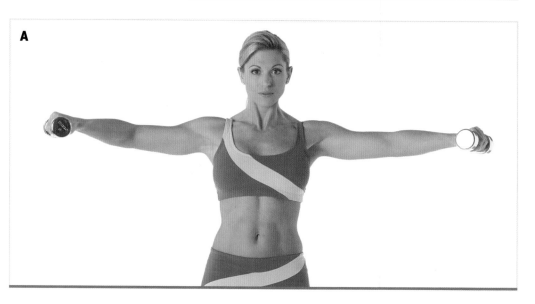

90-Degree Chest Fly

Muscles worked: Chest, shoulders (front, lateral, and rear deltoids), upper back

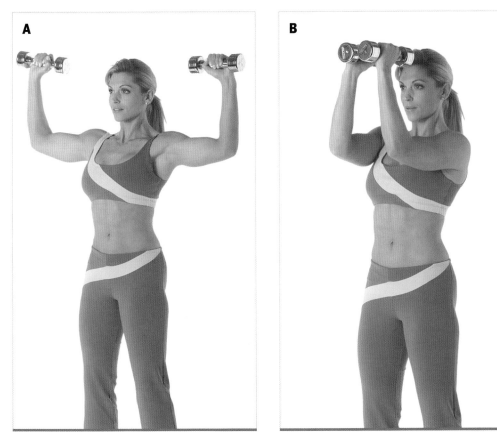

Beginner's Tip
Think about trying to touch your elbows together when doing this move to really squeeze the upper chest muscles.

A. Stand with your feet hip-width apart and your knees slightly bent, and hold a pair of dumbbells with your arms bent 90 degrees, elbows raised to shoulder height.

B. Squeeze your chest and bring your elbows together in front of your body at shoulder height. Open them back to the start and repeat.

Front Shoulder Raise

Muscles worked: Shoulders (front deltoids)

Beginner's Tip
For variety, try alternating arms instead of doing both at once. And remember not to use your back to lift the weights!

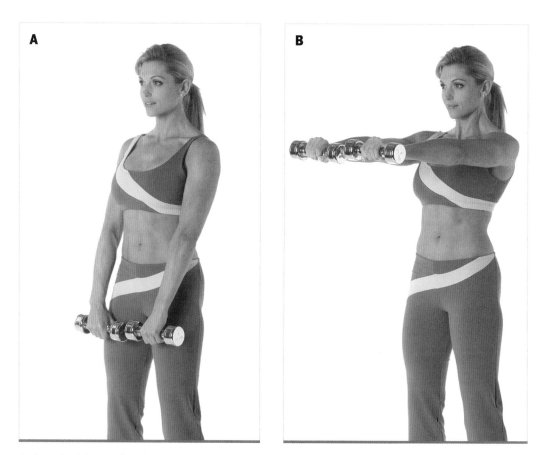

A. Stand with your feet hip-width apart and your knees slightly bent, and hold a pair of dumbbells in front of your thighs, palms facing your legs.

B. Slowly raise both weights in front of you to shoulder height, keeping your arms straight and your abs tight. Slowly lower the weights to the start and repeat right away.

Basic Reverse Lunge

Muscles worked: Quadriceps, hamstrings, glutes, calves

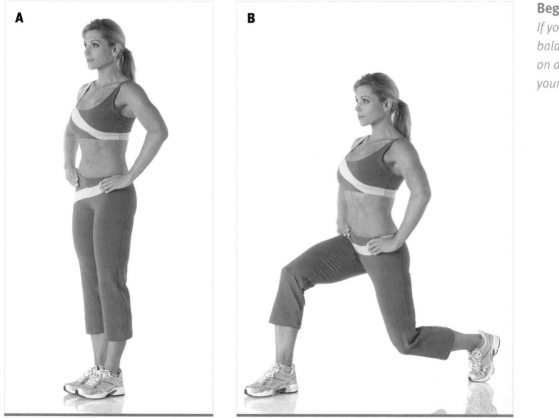

Beginner's Tip
If you're having trouble balancing, place a hand on a chair to stabilize yourself.

A. Stand with your feet and knees together, hands on your hips.

B. Take a large step backward onto the ball of one foot, balancing your weight between both legs. Your back heel should remain lifted off the floor. Bend both knees and lower your hips toward the floor until both your legs make 90-degree angles. Straighten your legs, stand back up to the start, and repeat.

Beginning Side Lunge

Muscles worked: Quadriceps, inner/outer thigh, glutes, hamstrings, calves

Beginner's Tip
A lot of people tend to lean forward when doing this move. Try to keep your torso upright as much as possible and bend through your knees and hips to lunge toward the floor.

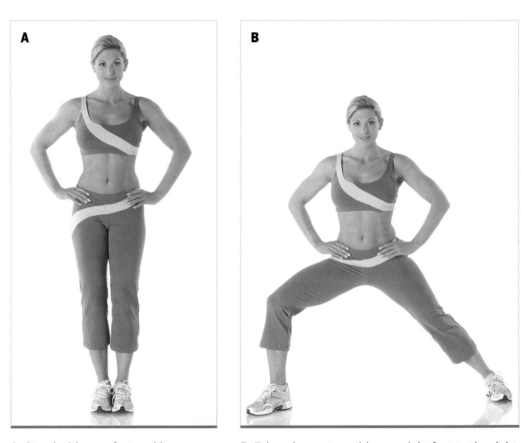

A. Stand with your feet and knees together, hands on your hips.

B. Take a large step with your right foot to the right side and lunge toward the floor. Make sure your right knee does not pass your right toe, and try to keep your entire left foot on the floor. Push off through your right foot to return to the start, and repeat, alternating sides.

Basic Squat

Muscles worked: Quadriceps, hamstrings, glutes, calves

Beginner's Tip

If you're having trouble with squatting form, practice using an actual chair. Place the rear legs of a chair against a wall for stability, then squat down and sit lightly in the chair, just barely touching your rear to the seat. Stand back up immediately and repeat.

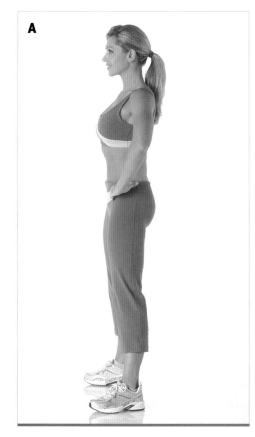

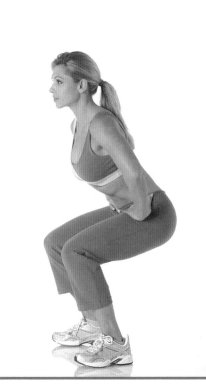

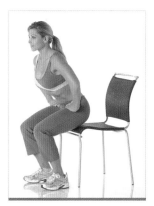

Use a chair to help you learn proper squatting form!

A. Stand with your feet hip-width apart and your hands on your hips.

B. Slowly squat toward the floor, bending your knees and kicking your hips back as if you were going to sit in a chair. When your thighs are almost parallel to the floor, or your heels begin to lift off the floor, stand back up to the start.

Ballet Squat

Muscles worked: Inner and outer thigh, quadriceps, hamstrings, glutes, calves

Beginner's Tip
Don't let your feet roll inward, as this affects the way your knees track over your toes. Keep your feet flat on the floor the whole time.

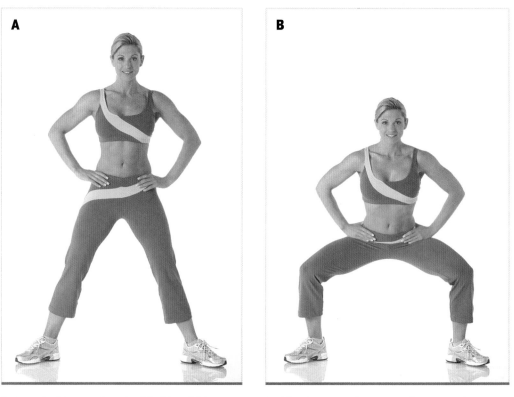

A. Stand with your feet double-hip-width apart and turn your legs out from the hip so your knees and toes are pointing on the diagonal.

B. Slowly squat down, tracking your knees over your toes and lowering until your thighs are parallel to the floor. Stand back up to the start, squeezing your glutes at the top, and go right into the next repetition.

Close Squat

Muscles worked: Quadriceps, glutes, hamstrings, calves

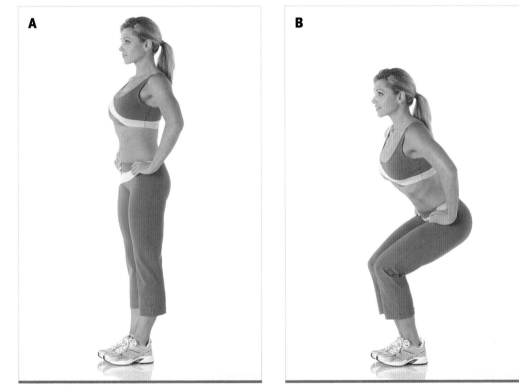

Beginner's Tip
Your weight should be in your heels for this move. If you can lift your toes off the floor when you're at the bottom of the squat, your weight is in your heels. If you can't, your weight is too far forward.

A. Stand with your feet and knees together, hands on your hips.

B. Slowly squat toward the floor, bending your knees and kicking your hips back as if you were sitting in a chair. Lower as far as possible without lifting your heels off the floor, then press through your heels to stand back up to the start.

Girly Push-up

Muscles worked: Chest, shoulders, triceps, abs, back

Beginner's Tip

If you need to rest at any point during the exercise, rest in the "up" position, with your arms extended and your abs tight (A). Hold here and breathe until you're ready for your next repetition.

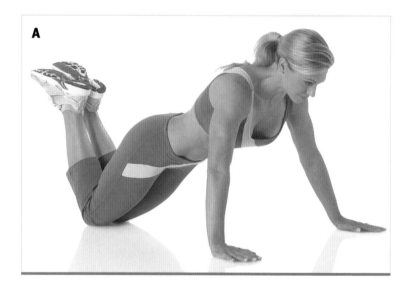

A. Kneel on the floor and place your hands wide on the ground outside your shoulders. Balance your weight between your hands and your knees, keeping your torso rigid and your abs tight.

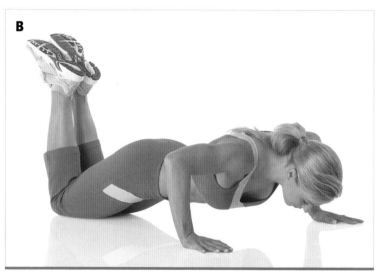

B. Bend your elbows to lower your torso almost to the floor, then press right back up to the start.

Beginning Superman

Muscles worked: Lower back, glutes

A. Lie facedown on the floor with your legs together. Make a cushion by stacking your hands on the floor and resting your forehead on top.

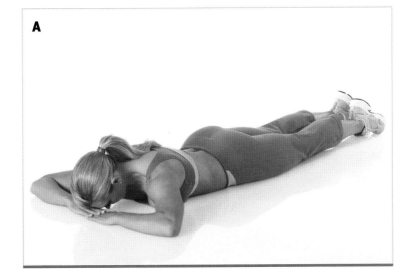

Beginner's Tip
As you improve, try to lift a little higher and hold a little longer each time you do this move.

B. Lift your torso and arms off the ground, keeping your head in line with your spine. Hold for two deep breaths, then lower back to the floor. Repeat.

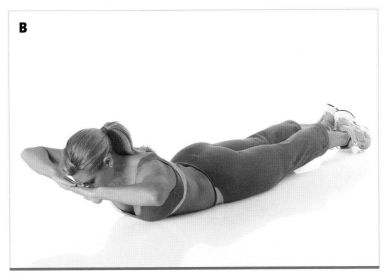

Half Plank

Muscles worked: Chest, shoulders, back, abs

Beginner's Tip
Don't let your butt sag! Keep your abs tight and your core steady. If you feel like your form is wavering during the move, lower to the floor, take a few breaths, then press back up and hold with the correct form.

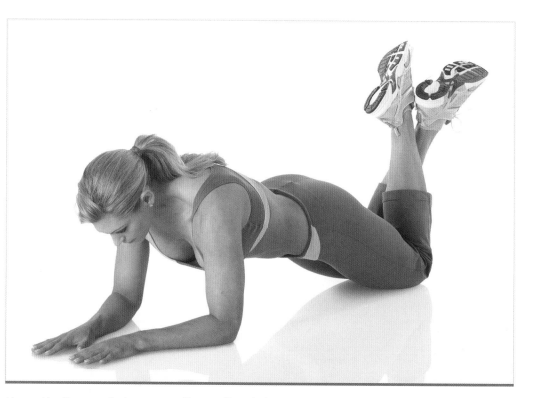

Lie on the floor and place your elbows directly beneath your shoulders, palms down. Bend your knees and cross your ankles above your legs. Lift your torso and hips off the floor so your head, shoulders, hips, and knees all form a straight line. Breathe and hold!

Donkey Kick

Muscles worked: Glutes, hamstrings, back, abs

A. Get on all fours with your hands directly underneath your shoulders and your knees directly underneath your hips, with one knee slightly lifted off the floor.

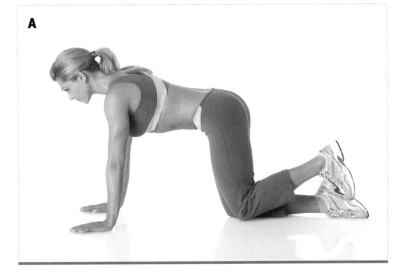

Beginner's Tip

This is not a high-kicking contest, and the height of your leg is less important than your form. If you feel like you're tipping to one side, lower your leg a bit to square your hips.

B. Lift one leg behind you with your knee bent and your foot flexed, pressing the sole of your shoe toward the ceiling. Your hips should remain square, hip-bones parallel to the floor. Slowly return your leg to the start and repeat right away. Do ten repetitions with one leg before switching to the other side. Alternate sides until your time runs out.

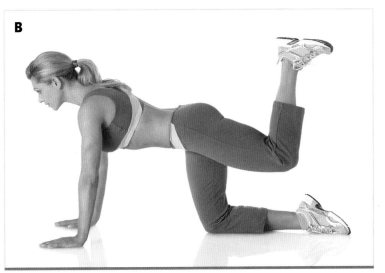

Side-Lying Leg Lift

Muscles worked: Outer thigh, glutes

Beginner's Tip
To really hit the outer hip, rotate your entire leg so your toes point straight ahead.

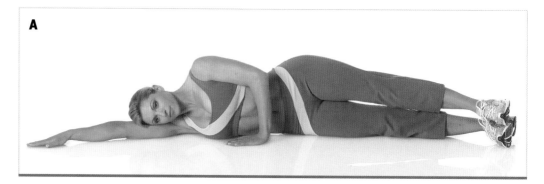

A. Lie on your side with your hips and knees stacked and your legs straight. Extend your arm along the floor and rest your head on this arm as if it's a cushion.

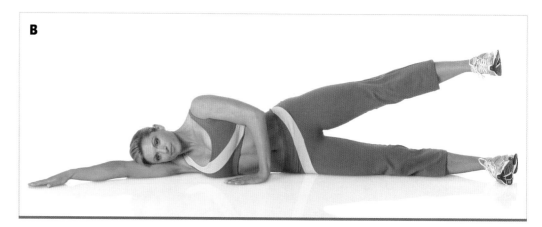

B. Slowly lift your top leg up toward the ceiling 12–18 inches. Hold for one count, then lower to the start.

Side-Lying Knee to Chest

Muscles worked: Outer thigh, glutes, quadriceps

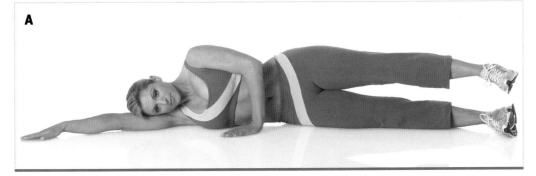

A. Lie on your side with your hips and knees stacked and your legs straight. Lift your top leg a few inches.

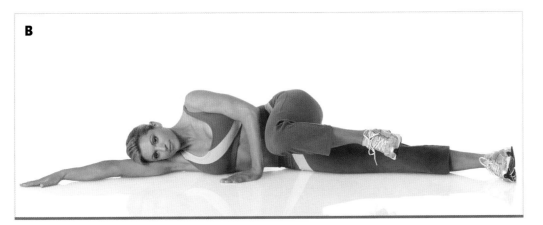

B. Bend your knee and bring it in toward your chest. Extend your leg back away from your chest, lower it to the start, and repeat.

Beginner's Tip
If you need more stability when doing this move, bend your bottom knee.

Basic Crunch

Muscles worked: Abs (rectus abdominus)

Beginner's Tip
If your neck aches, place the fingertips of both hands lightly behind your head to support it without pulling.

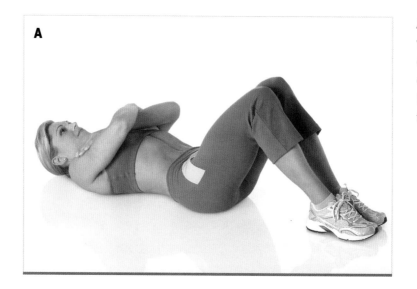

A. Lie on your back with your arms crossed over your chest, your knees bent, and your feet flat on the floor.

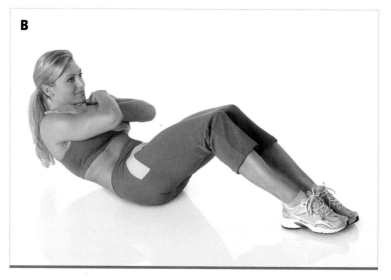

B. Exhale and slowly lift your head, shoulders, and upper back off the floor. Slowly lower to the start and repeat right away.

Ab Cycle

Muscles worked: Abs (rectus abdominus), obliques

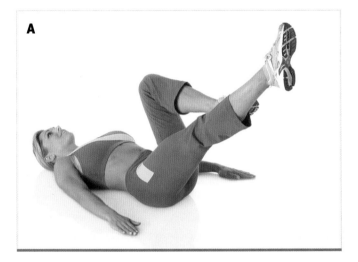

A

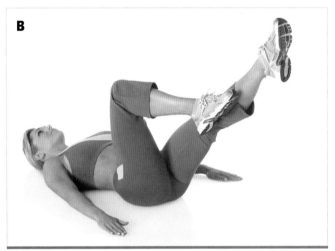

B

A. Lie on your back with your arms along your sides, and bend your knees, bringing them over your hips. Alternately extend one leg straight away from you while bringing the opposite knee toward your head.

B. Repeat in a rhythmic pattern.

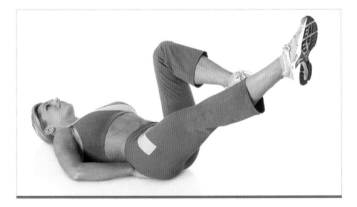

Note: If you have lower back problems, or feel pain in your lower back when doing this move, place your hands underneath your hips for additional support. Also extend your legs at a higher angle to decrease pressure on the back and hips and avoid excessive arching of the lower back.

Beginner's Tip
To change the difficulty of this move, change the angle at which you extend your legs: The closer to the floor you keep your legs, the harder it will be.

Bent-Over Row

Muscles worked: Back

Beginner's Tip
Stand sideways to a mirror when learning this move to make sure your back is flat and not rounded.

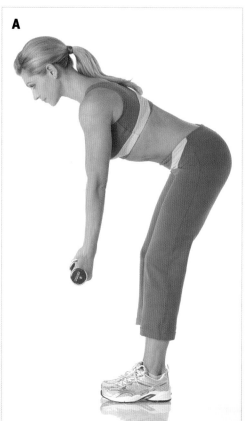

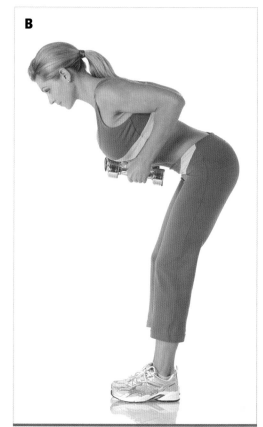

A. Stand with your feet together, knees slightly bent, and hold a pair of dumbbells at your sides. Bend forward from the waist so your torso is nearly parallel to the floor. Keep your back flat, and allow your arms to hang straight down from your shoulders, palms facing away from you.

B. Keep your torso steady and slowly pull the dumbbells toward your chest, leading with your elbows and keeping your arms in close to your sides. As you pull the weights up toward your body, rotate them slightly so that your palms are now facing each other. Slowly lower the weights back to the start.

Triceps Kickback

Muscles worked: Triceps

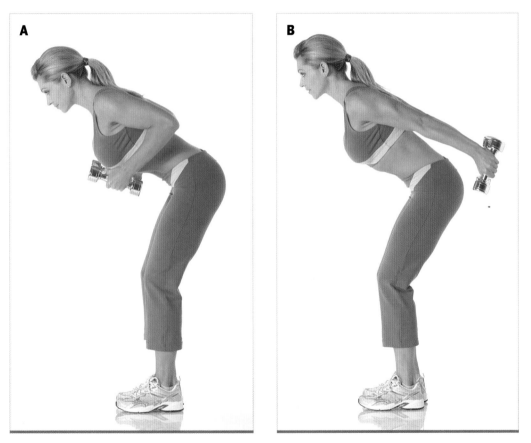

Beginner's Tip
To best isolate your triceps, imagine there is a long bolt running through your rib cage and pinning your elbows to your sides for this move.

A. Stand with your feet together, knees slightly bent, and hold a pair of dumbbells at your sides. Bend forward from your waist with a flat back so your torso is nearly parallel to the floor. Lift your elbows to come in line with your rib cage and pin them to your sides.

B. From here, extend your elbows and straighten your arms to press the dumbbells up and back. Bend your elbows to return to the start and repeat.

Half Jack

Muscles worked: Total body

Beginner's Tip
Land with your knees "soft" (i.e., bent slightly) at all times!

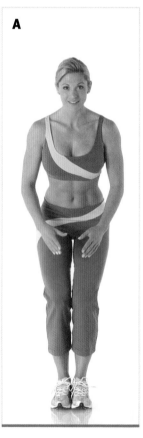

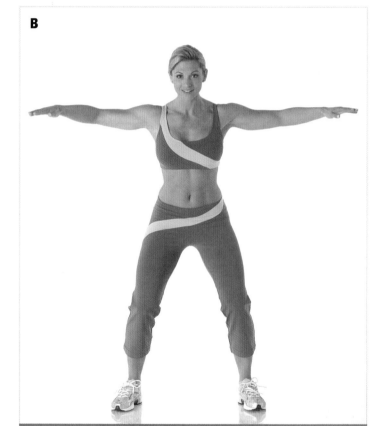

A. Stand with your feet and knees together, arms down.

B. Lightly jump your feet apart into a wide stance and bring your arms up to shoulder height. Jump back to the start and repeat in a rhythmic pattern.

Basic March

Muscles worked: Total body

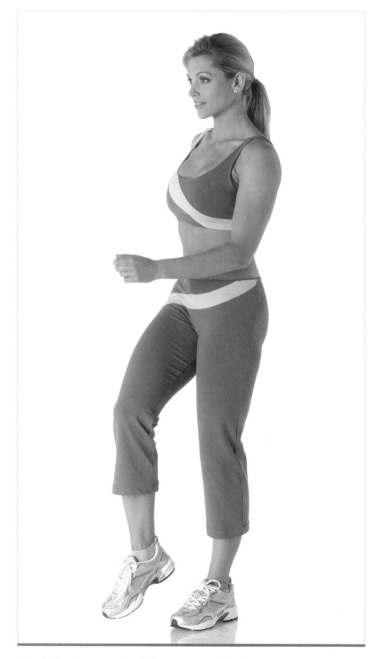

March in place, maintaining an even rhythm.

Beginner's Tip
Use your arms as well as your legs here to get the most out of this move.

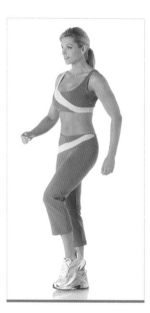

Step Touch

Muscles worked: Total body

Beginner's Tip
The more you bend your legs and the lower you get to the ground, the more work you'll put on your glutes!

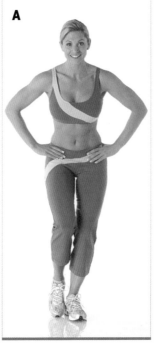

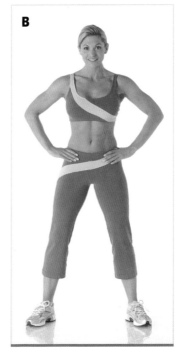

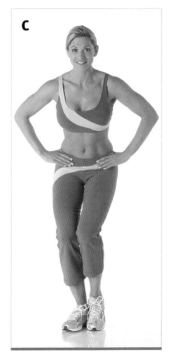

A. Stand with your feet together, knees slightly bent, hands on your hips. Tap your right toe next to your left foot.

B. Next, step with your right foot to the right side.

C. Now follow with your left, and touch your left toe down briefly next to your right foot. Next, step to the left with your left foot (B), and tap with your right (A). Repeat, alternating sides and using an even cadence.

Beginning Power Lunge

Muscles worked: Total body

Beginner's Tip

Don't let your front-lunging knee shoot past your front toe! Make your lunge go down instead of forward, keeping your front knee over your front toe to avoid injury.

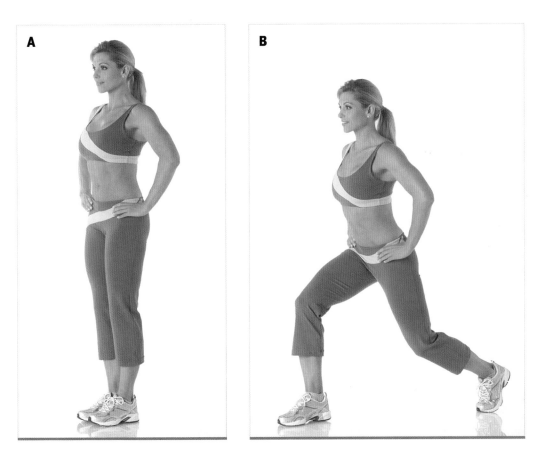

A. Stand with your feet together and your hands on your hips.

B. Take a giant step forward with your right foot, and lunge toward the floor. When your front leg makes a 90-degree angle, push off your front foot to return to the start. Repeat, alternating sides rhythmically.

Bunny Hop

Muscles worked: Total body

Beginner's Tip
Remember to land with your knees slightly bent to absorb the impact and avoid injury.

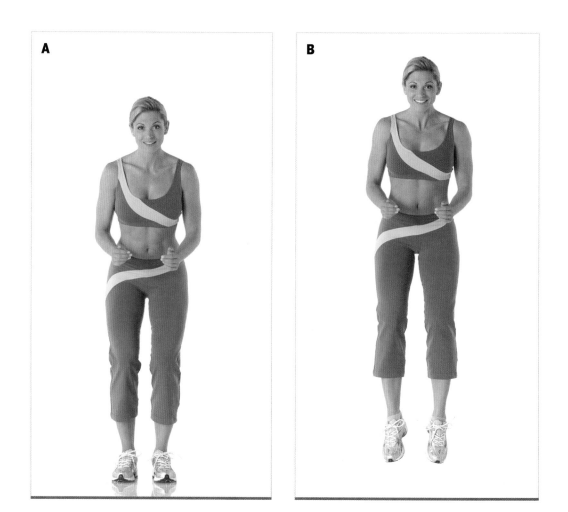

A. With your feet and knees slightly apart, hop up and down in place.

B. Maintain an even cadence, and use your arms to help you jump if needed.

Starter Speed Skate

Muscles worked: Total body

Beginner's Tip
Use the momentum of your arms to help carry you from side to side.

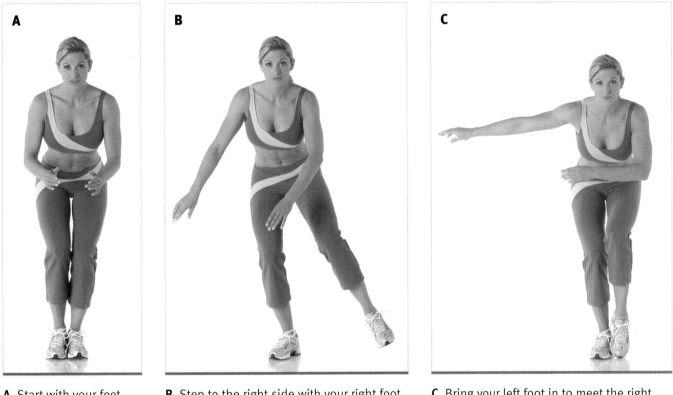

A. Start with your feet together, knees slightly bent, and bend forward slightly from the waist with your back flat and your abs tight.

B. Step to the right side with your right foot, simultaneously bringing your arms across your body to the right.

C. Bring your left foot in to meet the right, touching your left toe to the floor. Repeat, alternating sides.

Beginning Burpee

Muscles worked: Total body

Beginner's Tip
Keep your butt low and your abs tight when you're in the splayed (push-up) position (D).

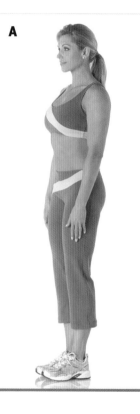

A. Stand with your feet together, knees slightly bent, arms at your sides.

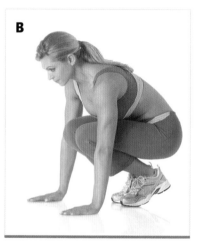

B. Bend your knees to crouch toward the floor, placing your hands flat on the ground in front of you, spaced about a foot apart.

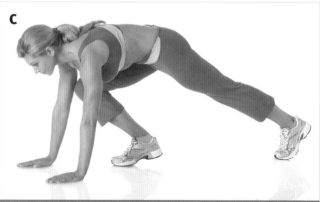

C. Step back behind you with one foot.

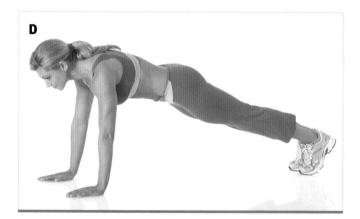

D. Follow with the other foot. You should now be in a push-up position. Step your feet back underneath your hips one at a time to come back to a crouch position (B), then stand up to complete one repetition. Repeat sequence.

Level I Suggested Schedule

WEEK	MONDAY	TUESDAY	WEDNESDAY	THURSDAY	FRIDAY	SATURDAY	SUNDAY
1	Circuit 1	Trouble Spots	Rest	Circuit 2	Rest	Lower Body/Cardio	Rest
2	Circuit 1	Trouble Spots	Rest	Circuit 2	Rest	Lower Body/Cardio	Rest
3	Circuit 1	Trouble Spots	Rest	Circuit 2	Optional Cardio (20 minutes)	Lower Body/Cardio	Rest
4	Circuit 1	Trouble Spots	Rest	Circuit 2	Optional Cardio (20 minutes)	Lower Body/Cardio	Rest

Week 1: Do each circuit once.
Week 2: Do each circuit once or twice.

Week 3: Do each circuit twice.
Week 4: Do each circuit twice or three times.

CIRCUIT 1

1. Biceps Curl
2. Beginning Power Lunge
3. Overhead Triceps Extension
4. Basic Squat
5. Upright Row
6. Basic Reverse Lunge
7. Bent-Over Row
8. Bunny Hop
9. Overhead Shoulder Press
10. Half Jack

CIRCUIT 2

1. Strongman Curl
2. Starter Speed Skate
3. Triceps Kickback
4. Beginning Burpee
5. Lateral Shoulder Raise
6. Ballet Squat
7. 90-Degree Chest Fly
8. Close Squat
9. Front Shoulder Raise
10. Basic March

LOWER BODY/CARDIO

1. Basic March
2. Step Touch
3. Basic Squat
4. Beginning Side Lunge
5. Close Squat
6. Beginning Power Lunge
7. Bunny Hop
8. Starter Speed Skate
9. Beginning Burpee
10. Half Jack

TROUBLE SPOTS WORKOUT

1. Girly Push-up
2. Beginning Superman
3. Half Plank
4. Donkey Kick
5. Side-Lying Leg Lift—Right Side
6. Side-Lying Knee to Chest—Right Side
7. Side-Lying Leg Lift—Left Side
8. Side-Lying Knee to Chest—Left Side
9. Basic Crunch
10. Ab Cycle

LEVEL II

Welcome to Level II! By now, you're getting stronger and need more of a challenge. In Level II you'll take the basics you learned in Level I and combine them into "double moves." In addition, you'll be increasing the intensity of the Lower-Body/Cardio moves to burn more calories and get more fit.

Level II Instructions

Points of Focus
- pacing yourself
- performing slow, controlled repetitions
- using proper form
- using full range of motion
- learning double movement patterns for basic exercises
- warming up and cooling down properly

Who Is This Level For?

Anyone who is comfortable with all the moves in Level I and is ready for a new challenge. The "double moves" take a little more thought and practice, testing your body and your brain alike.

NOTABLE NOTES

Next to many of the move names, you'll notice additional information. For example, next to Double-Duty Delts you'll see Front Shoulder Raise/Lateral Shoulder Raise. This means that Double-Duty Delts is a combination of two basic shoulder moves: front shoulder raises and lateral shoulder raises. If you forget the form of a particular basic movement, look it up in Level I.

During your lower-body and Lower-Body/Cardio exercises, I encourage you add some arm movements to bump up the calorie burn. Don't be regimented—go freestyle! Do chest presses, punches, lateral raises, jazz hands—have fun with it!

Circuit Works

1. Try to do each move for 30–45 seconds, starting with 30 seconds per move and working your way up to 45 seconds as you get stronger.
2. Because you've built a solid base of endurance in Level I, cut your rest time between sets to 45 seconds for all workouts.
3. Go through each circuit at least once the first week, twice if you're feeling strong. By the end of the month, you should be doing each circuit three times through.

Circuit Math

   10 moves @ 45 seconds each
+ 45 seconds rest in between moves
= 15 minutes each circuit (once through)

Which Weights?

Double moves are significantly harder than single moves, so for the first few weeks of Level II, choose lighter dumbbells so you don't burn out quickly. As you get used to the moves and increase your strength, increase your dumbbell weight accordingly.

Cardio Rx

Do at least 30–40 continuous minutes of cardio for your workouts this month.

Good Level II Cardio Ideas
- power walking or jogging outside
- elliptical trainer with arms
- Stairmaster
- hill walking
- treadmill walking on an incline (3–6 percent)
- stationary biking or beginning Spinning classes
- in-line skating

Bi-Row (Biceps Curl / Upright Row)

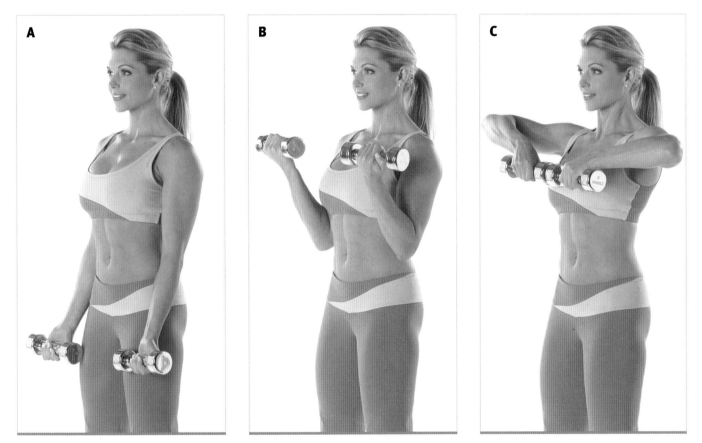

A. Stand with your feet hip-width apart and your knees slightly bent, and hold a pair of dumbbells in front of your thighs, palms facing up.

B. Lift the weights in a biceps curl, keeping your elbows in tight to your body.

C. Lower the weights to the start, then turn your palms to face your thighs and lift the dumbbells up toward your chin in an upright row, leading the motion with your elbows and keeping your shoulders down and back. Repeat, alternating moves.

Uptown Arms (Overhead Front Raise / Overhead Triceps Extension)

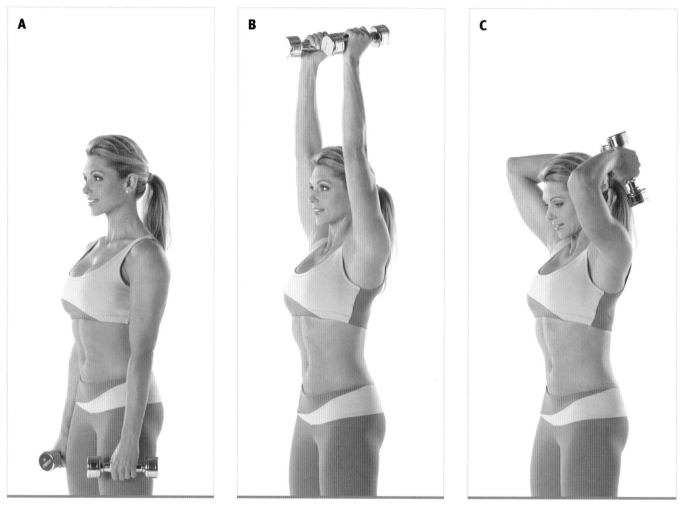

A. Stand with your feet hip-width apart and hold a pair of dumbbells at your sides, palms facing each other.

B. Slowly raise the weights in a large arc in front of your body, lifting them all the way up to an overhead position, arms close to your ears.

C. From here, bend your elbows and drop the weights behind your head in a triceps extension. Straighten your arms (B), then reverse the arc to return to the start (A).

Double-Duty Delts (Front Shoulder Raise / Lateral Shoulder Raise)

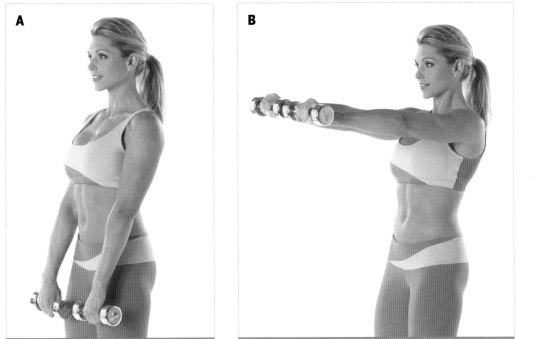

A. Stand with your feet hip-width apart and your knees slightly bent, and hold a pair of dumbbells in front of your thighs, palms facing your legs.

B. Slowly raise the weights to shoulder height in a front shoulder raise.

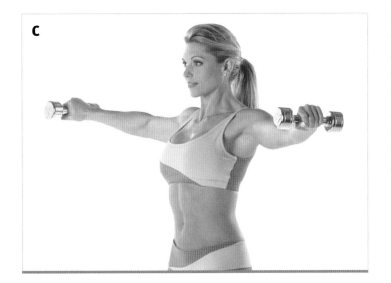

C. Lower to the start (A), then bend your elbows slightly and lift the weights up and out to the sides in a lateral raise, leading the motion with your elbows. Lower to the start. Repeat, alternating moves.

Back to Business (Bent-Over Row / Rear Shoulder Fly)

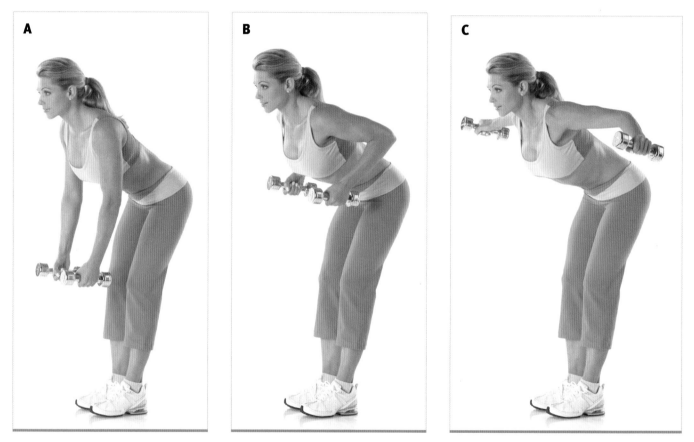

A. Stand with your feet hip-width apart and your knees slightly bent, and hold a pair of dumbbells at your sides. Bend forward from your waist, keeping your back flat, until your torso is nearly parallel to the floor. Allow your arms to hang straight down from your shoulders, palms facing each other.

B. Keeping your torso steady, slowly pull the dumbbells toward your chest in a bent-over row, keeping your arms in close to your sides.

C. Lower the weights to the start (A), then raise them up and out to the sides in a rear shoulder fly, keeping your hands in your peripheral vision and raising them to shoulder height. Lower to the start and repeat, alternating moves.

Fly Like an Eagle (Overhead Shoulder Press / 90-Degree Chest Fly)

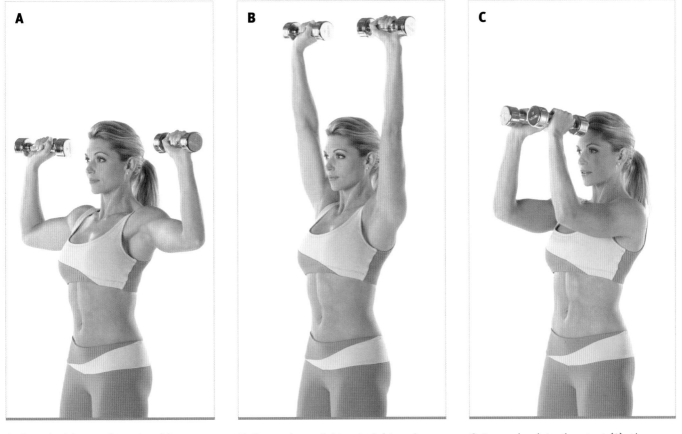

A. Stand with your feet shoulder-width apart and your knees slightly bent, and hold a pair of dumbbells at ear height, palms facing forward, wrists stacked over your elbows, and elbows raised to shoulder height.

B. Press the weights straight up in an overhead shoulder press until your arms reach full extension.

C. Lower back to the start (A), then bring your elbows together in front of your head at shoulder height in a 90-degree chest fly. Open your arms back to the start and repeat, alternating moves.

Fly-Girl Curls (Biceps Strongman Curl / Straight-Arm Chest Fly)

A. Stand with your feet hip-width apart and your knees slightly bent. Hold a pair of dumbbells at shoulder height, your arms held straight out and parallel to the floor, and your palms facing the ceiling.

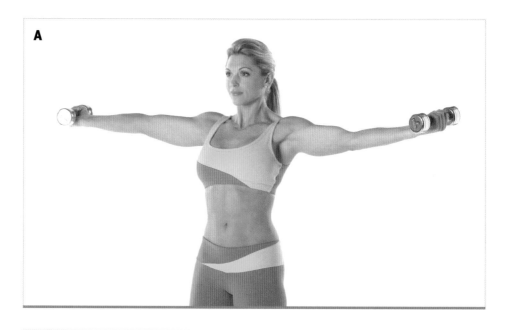

B. Curl the dumbbells in toward your head in a strongman curl, then extend back to the start (A).

C. Keeping your arms straight, turn your palms to face front, then bring your hands together in front of your chest at shoulder height. Open back to the start and repeat, alternating moves.

Note: You may want to use lighter dumbbells for this move initially. It's difficult to keep your weights elevated like this for an extended period of time!

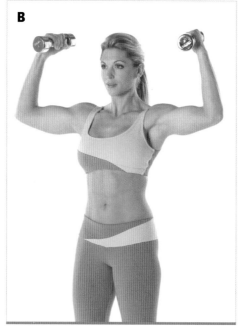

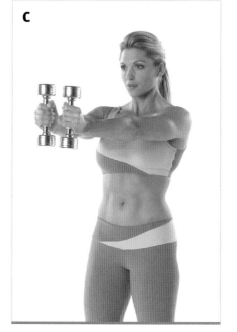

Circle T

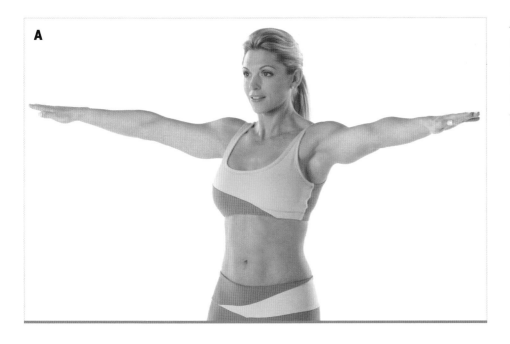

A. Stand with your feet hip-width apart and your knees slightly bent, and raise your arms to the sides in line with your shoulders, parallel to the floor, to make a T with your body, palms facing the floor.

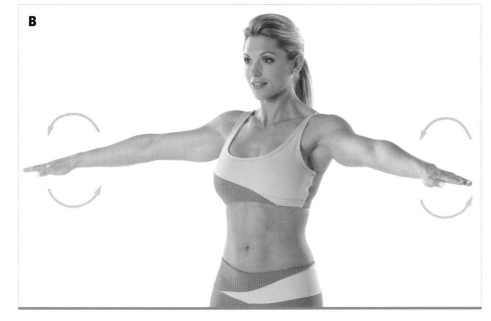

B. Draw small circles in the air with your arms, keeping them at shoulder height. Change directions every 15 repetitions.

Shoulder T (Front Shoulder Raise / Straight-Arm Chest Fly)

A. Stand with your feet hip-width apart and your knees slightly bent, and hold a pair of dumbbells, palms facing your thighs.

B. Raise the weights to shoulder height in front of your body.

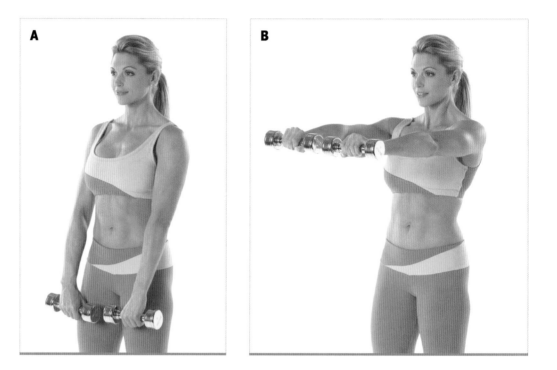

C. Next, open them out to the sides to make a T. Bring your arms back together in front of your chest (B), then lower to the start (A) to complete one repetition.

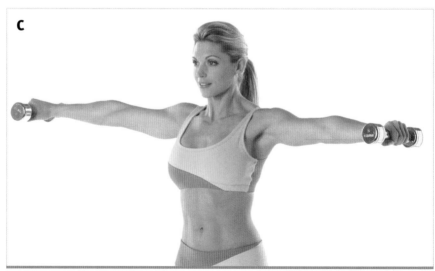

Soccer Squat (Basic Squat / Inner Thigh)

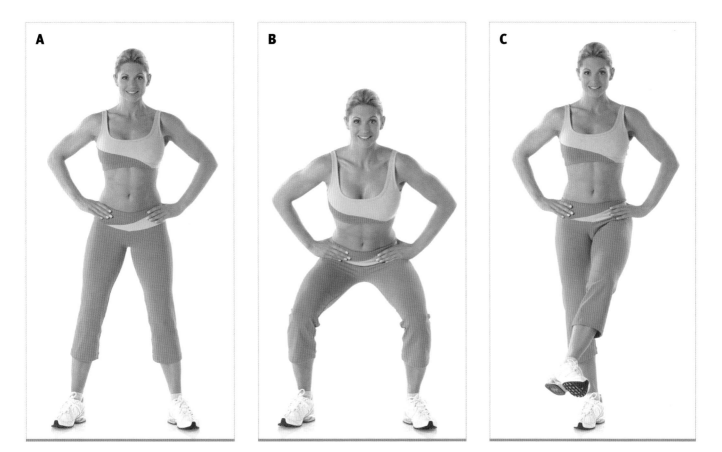

A. Stand with your feet shoulder-width apart, knees slightly bent.

B. Do a slow basic squat, kicking your hips back as if you were sitting in a chair.

C. Stand back up to the start and kick an imaginary soccer ball across your body to the front, leading the kick with the inside of your foot. Replace your foot, do another squat, and repeat, kicking with alternate sides.

High-Knee Reverse Lunge

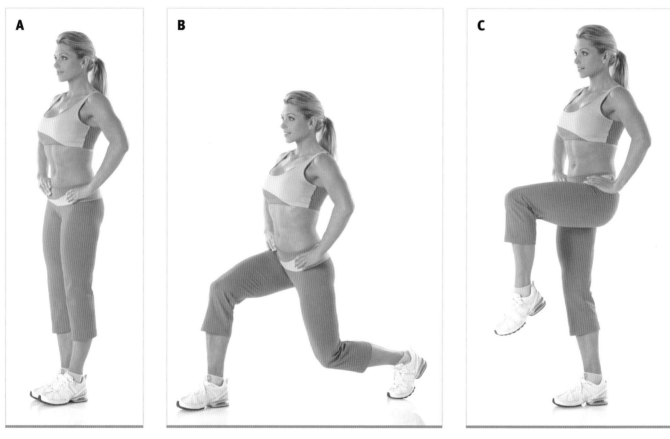

A. Stand with your feet together, hands on your hips.

B. Take a large step backward onto the ball of your left foot in a reverse lunge, lowering until your right thigh is nearly parallel to the floor.

C. Push off your left foot, straighten your right leg, then bring your left leg through to the front of your body, lifting your left knee to hip height. Step back with the left foot into another reverse lunge (B), then return to the start (A). Repeat on the other leg.

Ballet Squat Plus (Ballet Squat / Calf Raise)

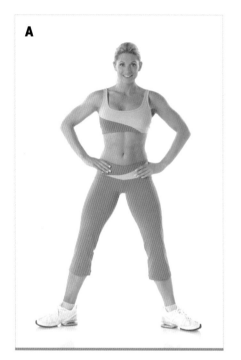

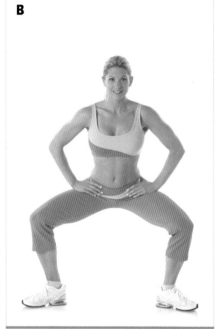

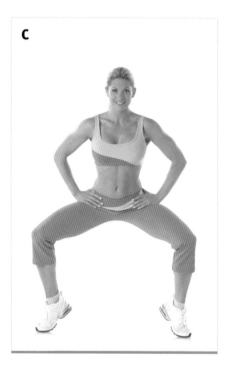

A. Stand with your feet double hip–width apart and turn your legs out from the hip so your knees and toes are pointing on the diagonal.

B. Do a slow ballet squat, tracking your knees over your toes and keeping your feet flat on the floor.

C. When your thighs are nearly parallel to the floor, pause and lift your heels off the floor in a calf raise. Lower your heels and stand back up to the start to complete one repetition. Repeat sequence.

Squat Plus (Close Squat / Knee Raise)

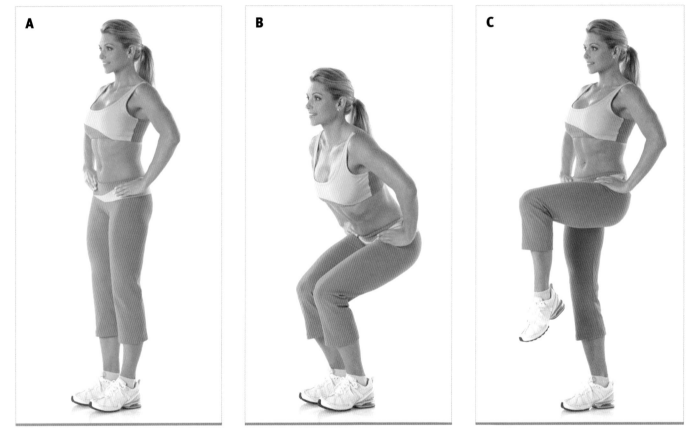

A. Stand with your feet and knees together, hands on your hips.

B. Do a slow close squat by bending your knees and kicking your hips back as if you were sitting in a chair.

C. As you stand back to the start, lift one knee to the front of your body at hip height. Put your foot back down, do another close squat, then lift the opposite knee to the front. Continue this way, alternating knees.

Open and Close Squat (Basic Squat / Close Squat)

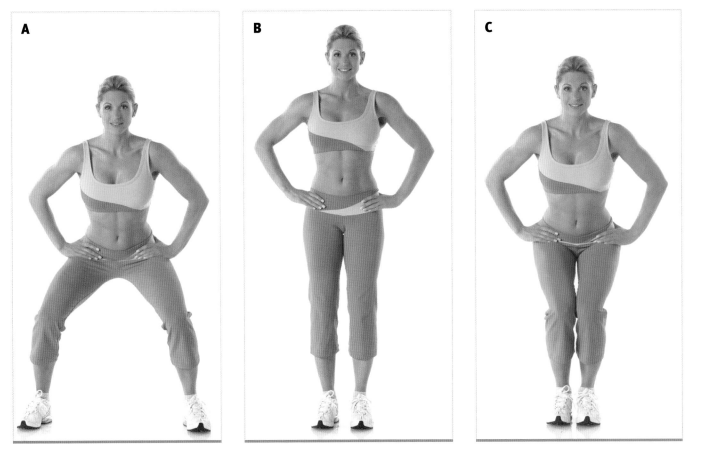

A. Stand with your feet and knees slightly wider than shoulder-width apart, hands on your hips. Do a slow basic squat by bending your knees and kicking your hips back as if you were sitting in a chair.

B. Stand up and step your feet together.

C. Do one repetition of a close squat. Repeat, alternating moves.

Side Lunge 'n' Lift (Side Lunge / Abductor Lift)

A. Stand with your feet and knees together, hands on your hips.

B. Take a large step with your right foot and lower into a right side lunge.

C. Push off your right foot and balance on your left leg as you simultaneously lift your right leg up and out to the side of your body. Return to the start. Repeat, alternating sides.

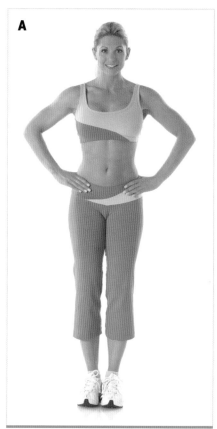

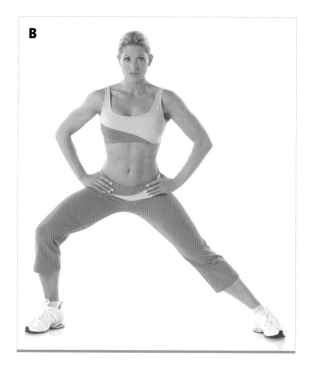

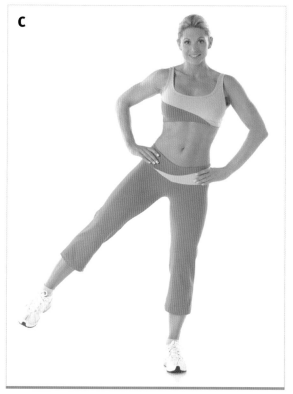

Kick 'n' Row (Triceps Kickback / Bent-Over Row)

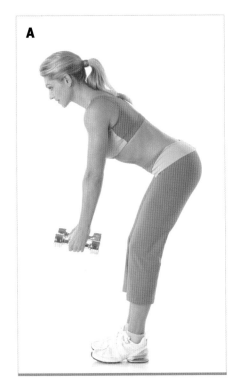

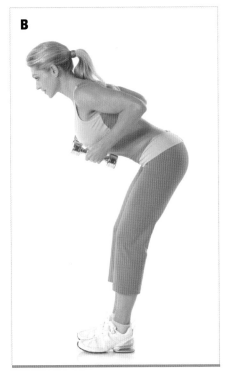

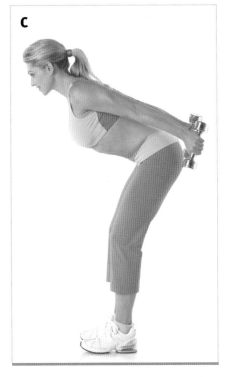

A. Stand with your feet hip-width apart and your knees slightly bent, and hold a pair of dumbbells at your sides. Bend forward from your waist, keeping your back flat, until your torso is nearly parallel to the floor.

B. Pull the weights in to your chest in a bent-over row.

C. Next, pin your elbows to your sides and straighten your elbows to extend your arms in a triceps kickback. Reverse the motion by bending your elbows once more (B), then extending your arms toward the floor (A).

Tough-Girl Push-up

A. Place both hands flat on the floor outside your shoulders, and extend your legs behind you, keeping your knees and feet together. Balance your weight between your hands and your toes, and tighten your abs and glutes to stabilize your torso. Your head, shoulders, hips, and heels should all be in one line.

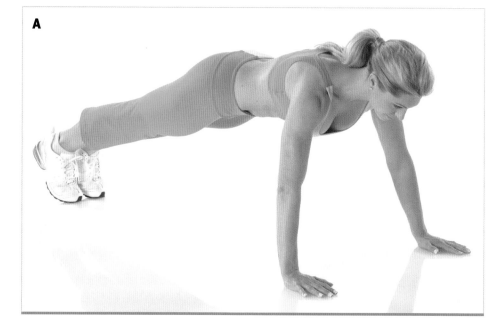

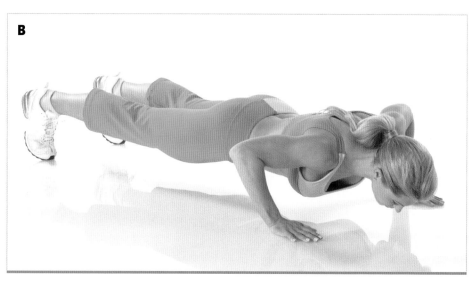

B. Maintain this position as you bend your elbows to lower your torso toward the floor. When your chest nearly touches the floor, press back up to the start. Repeat, resting in the "up" position when necessary.

Superman

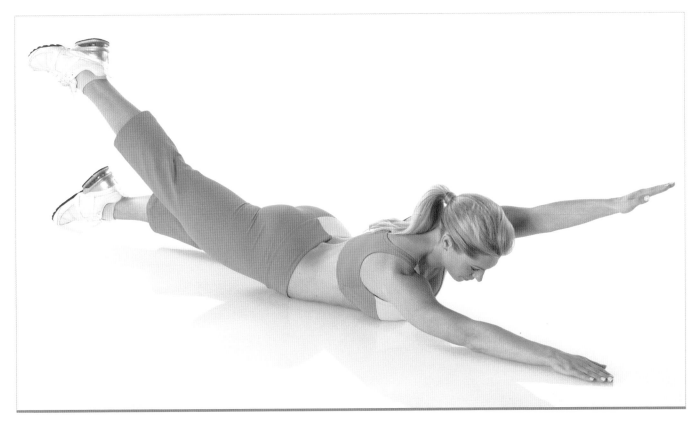

Lie facedown on the floor with your legs together and your arms stretched overhead along the floor. Simultaneously raise one leg and the opposite arm off the floor and hold for two deep breaths. Lower to the start and repeat, alternating sides.

Plank

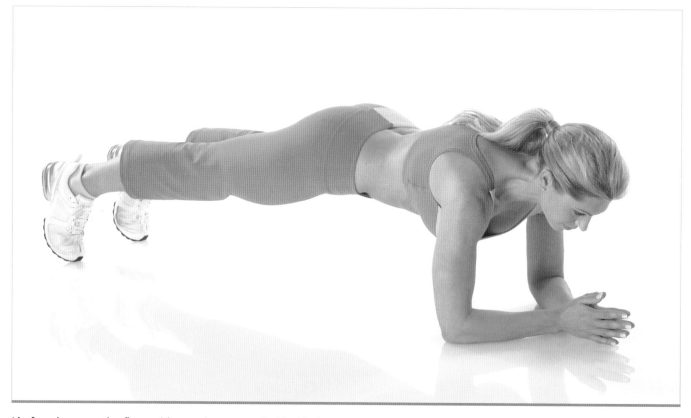

Lie facedown on the floor with your legs extended behind you. Line your elbows up underneath your shoulders and press your palms together underneath your chin. Turn your toes under and lift your torso, hips, and thighs off the floor, balancing your weight between your forearms and your toes, and tightening your abs and glutes for stability. Your head, shoulders, hips, and heels should all be in one line. Breathe deeply and hold this position for as long as you can. To take a break, simply drop your knees to the floor a moment, then raise yourself back up into position again.

Straight-Leg Donkey Kick

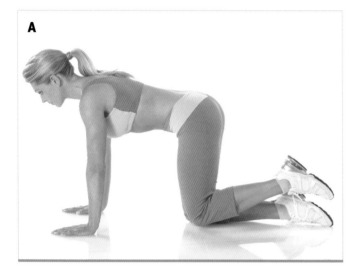

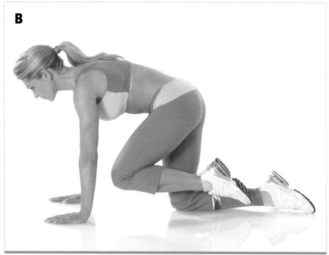

A. Get on all fours with your hands directly underneath your shoulders and your knees directly underneath your hips, one knee lifted off the floor.

B. Bring the lifted knee in toward your chest.

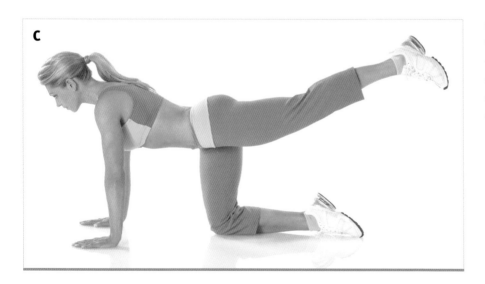

C. Next, extend it straight out behind you, lifting it slightly toward the ceiling while keeping your hips square. Bend your knee, bringing it once more into your chest (B), replace it on the floor, then repeat on the other side.

Side Plank

A. Lie on your left side with your left elbow placed underneath your left shoulder. Extend your legs away from you, hips and feet stacked, right hand on your hip.

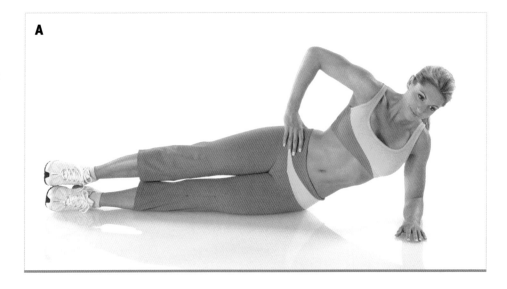

A

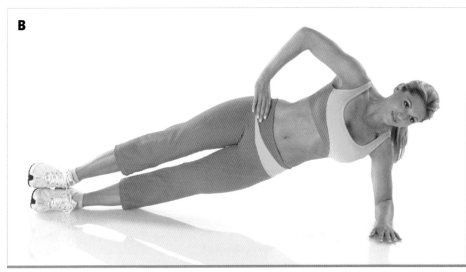

B

B. Lift your hips so your body makes a straight line through your shoulder, hip, knee, and ankle. Hold here and breathe. Repeat on the other side.

Get Hip (Side-Lying Leg Lift / Side-Lying Knee to Chest)

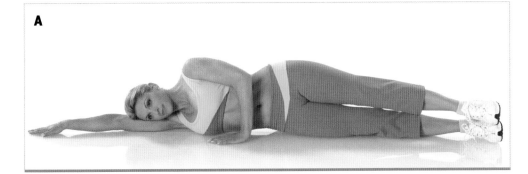

A. Lie on your side with your hips and knees stacked.

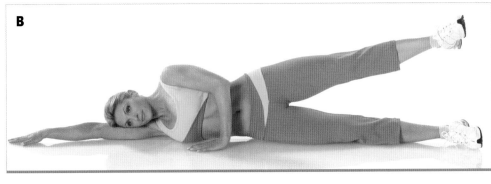

B. Slowly lift your top leg up toward the ceiling in a side-lying leg lift.

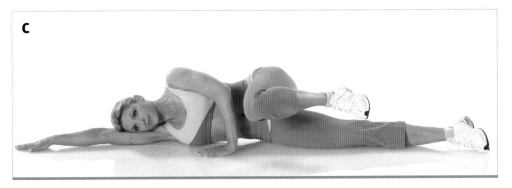

C. Lower almost to the start, then bend your knee and bring it in toward your chest. Extend your leg and repeat, rolling over and alternating sides every 10 repetitions.

Bridge

A. Lie on your back with your arms along your sides, your knees bent, and your feet flat on the floor, about 12 inches apart.

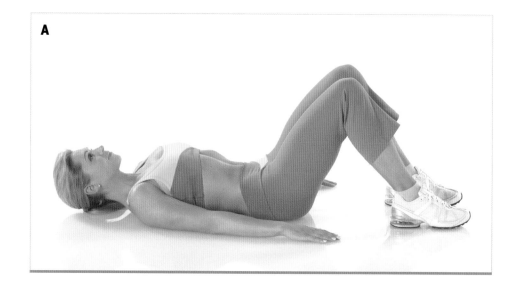

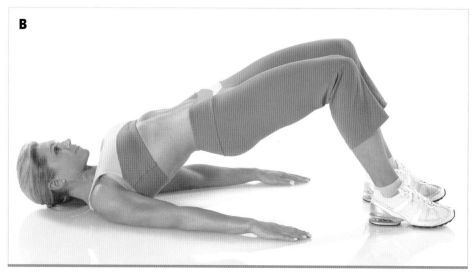

B. Squeeze your glutes and hamstrings to lift your hips into the air, so your knees, hips, and shoulders all come in line. Hold briefly, then lower to the start and repeat.

Feet-Up Crunch

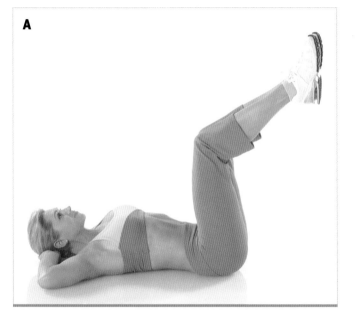

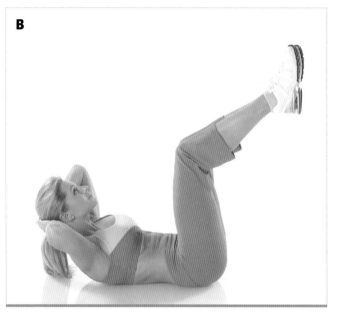

A. Lie on your back with your hands behind your head, fingertips touching but not laced, your knees bent, and your legs lifted over your hips.

B. Slowly lift your head, shoulders, and upper back off the floor, keeping your chin lifted off your chest and your elbows out to the sides. Hold briefly, then uncurl, return to the start, and repeat right away.

Half Power Lunge

A. Stand with your feet together and your hands on your hips.

B. Bend your knees and hop your feet apart, landing with your right foot forward and your left foot back, knees bent.

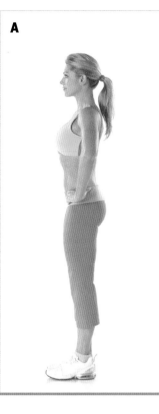

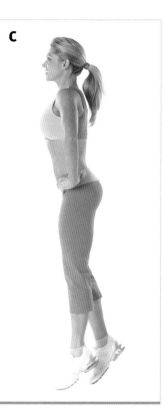

C. Hop into the air and switch feet

D. Land with your left foot forward and your right foot back, knees bent. Repeat, alternating sides rhythmically.

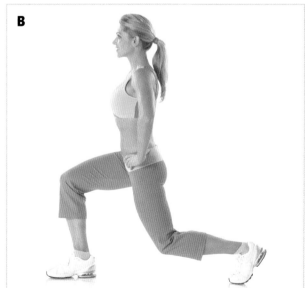

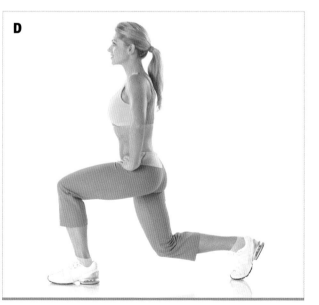

Ski Hop

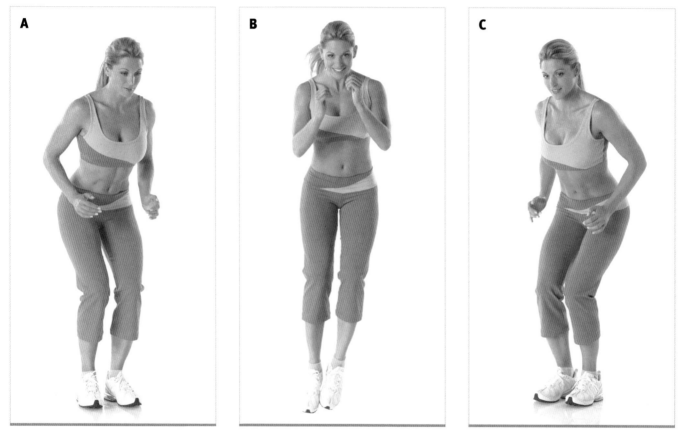

A. With your feet and knees together, do a series of small jumps from side to side.

B. Imagine you're jumping over an invisible line on the ground, landing with your knees bent every time.

C. Add a little twist in there as well, as if you're really skiing down a mountainside!

Jump Around the Clock

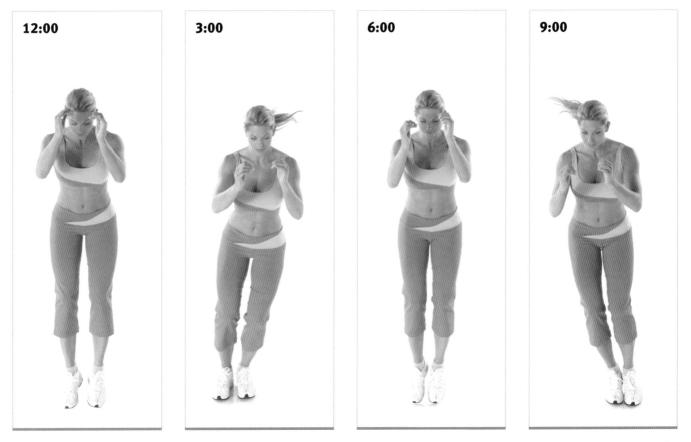

| 12:00 | 3:00 | 6:00 | 9:00 |

Stand with your feet and knees together, and imagine you're standing in the middle of a giant clock face. Jump with both feet to the 12 (directly in front of you), then back to the center. Then jump to the 3 (to your right) and back to the center. Continue this pattern for the 6 (behind you) and the 9 (to your left). Repeat, alternating clockwise and counterclockwise directions.

Full Jack

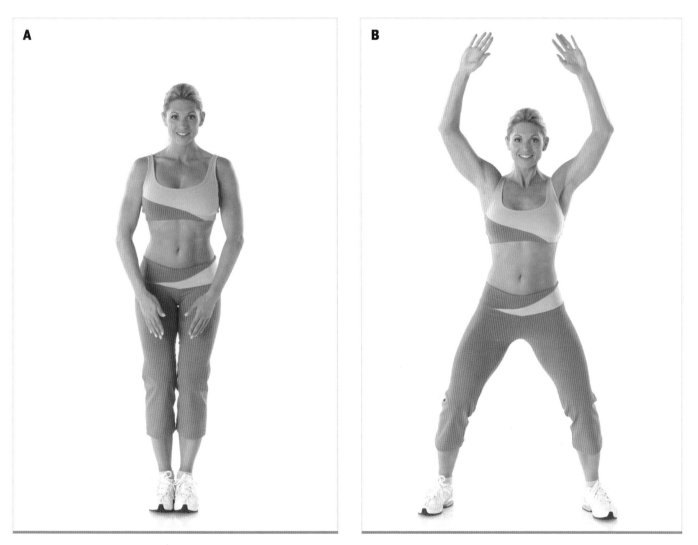

A. Stand with your feet and knees together and your hands in front of your thighs.

B. Lightly jump your feet apart into a wide stance and raise your arms completely overhead. Immediately jump back to the start and repeat in a rhythmic pattern, landing each time with your knees slightly bent.

Speed Skate

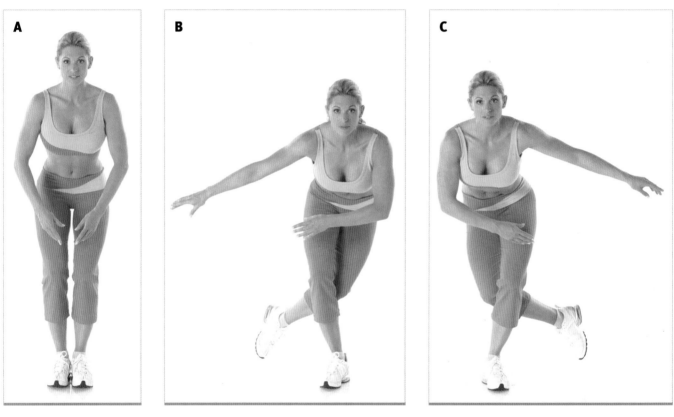

A. Stand with your feet together and your hands in front of your thighs. Bend forward slightly from the waist, keeping your abs tight and your back flat.

B. Hop to the right side with your right foot and bring your arms across your body to the right. Bring your left foot behind your right leg instead of touching it to the floor.

C. Now hop to the left, and bring your right leg behind your left, sweeping your arms across your body to the left. Repeat rhythmically, alternating sides.

Knees-Up March

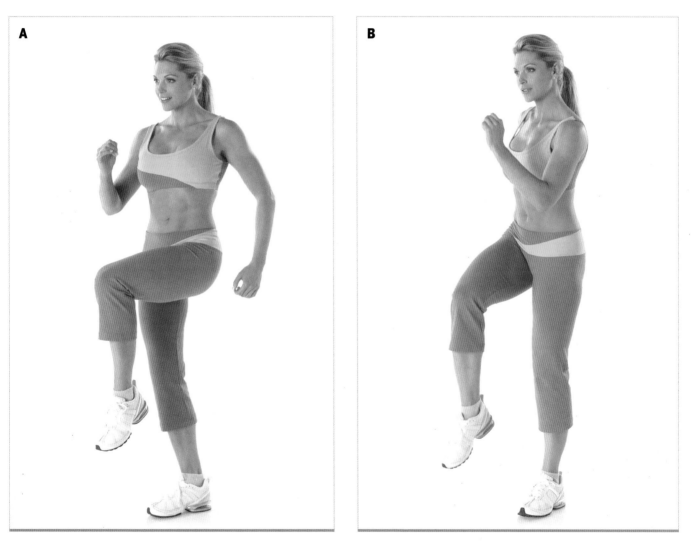

A. March in place, alternately bringing one knee up to hip height.

B. Pump your arms in opposition.

Burpee

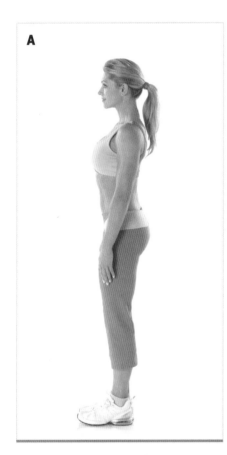

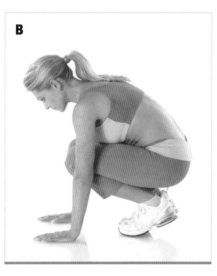

B. Crouch down, placing your hands flat on the floor in front of you, spaced about a foot apart.

C. Hop both feet behind you simultaneously, bringing your body into a push-up position. Hold briefly, then hop both feet back underneath your hips in a crouch position (B), and stand back up to the start to complete one repetition. Repeat sequence.

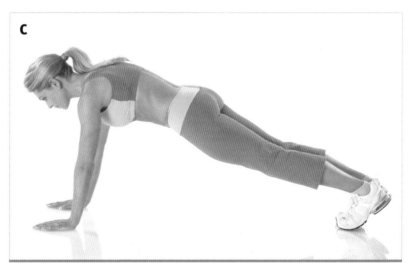

A. Stand with your feet hip-width apart, your knees slightly bent, and your arms at your sides.

Level II Suggested Schedule

WEEK	MONDAY	TUESDAY	WEDNESDAY	THURSDAY	FRIDAY	SATURDAY	SUNDAY
1	Circuit 1 and Trouble Spots	Lower Body/Cardio	Rest	Circuit 2	Cardio (30 minutes)	Rest or Lower Body/Cardio	Rest
2	Circuit 1 and Trouble Spots	Lower Body/Cardio	Rest	Circuit 2	Cardio (30–35 minutes)	Rest or Lower Body/Cardio	Rest
3	Circuit 1	Lower Body/Cardio	Rest	Circuit 2 and Trouble Spots	Cardio (35–40 minutes)	Rest or Lower Body/Cardio	Rest
4	Circuit 1	Lower Body/Cardio	Rest	Circuit 2 and Trouble Spots	Cardio (35–40 minutes)	Rest or Lower Body/Cardio	Rest

Week 1: Do each circuit once or twice.
Week 2: Do each circuit twice.

Week 3: Do each circuit twice or three times.
Week 4: Do each circuit three times.

CIRCUIT 1
1. Bi-Row
2. Half Power Lunge
3. Uptown Arms
4. Soccer Squat
5. Double-Duty Delts
6. High-Knee Reverse Lunge
7. Back to Business
8. Ski Hop
9. Fly Like an Eagle
10. Full Jack

LOWER BODY/CARDIO
1. Knees-Up March
2. Ski Hop
3. Open and Close Squat
4. Side Lunge 'n' Lift
5. Squat Plus
6. Half Power Lunge
7. Jump Around the Clock
8. Speed Skate
9. Burpee
10. Full Jack

CIRCUIT 2
1. Fly-Girl Curls
2. Speed Skate
3. Kick 'n' Row
4. Burpee
5. Circle T
6. Ballet Squat Plus
7. Shoulder T
8. Squat Plus
9. Uptown Arms
10. Knees-Up March

TROUBLE SPOTS WORKOUT
1. Tough-Girl Push-up
2. Superman
3. Plank
4. Straight-Leg Donkey Kick
5. Side Plank—Right Side
6. Get Hip—Right Side
7. Side Plank—Left Side
8. Get Hip—Left Side
9. Bridge
10. Feet-Up Crunch

LEVEL III

Welcome to your Level III workouts! Those of you who have reached this point should be very proud of yourselves. You're getting fit and strong and are doing great! Here in Level III, you'll be learning "triple moves," where you'll take the combinations from Level II and add an element of balance, stability, or core strength to each one. You'll also increase the intensity of the lower-body and cardio moves significantly for an excellent total-body workout!

Now, I'm not going to lie: Level III is challenging, but I know you can do it! There is nothing radically new in here. You've already done most of the moves at least once in the past 8 weeks; now it's time to turn up the intensity!

Level III Instructions

Points of Focus
• coordination and balance
• using proper form
• using full range of motion
• learning triple-movement patterns
• landing with soft knees during cardio moves
• warming up and cooling down properly

Who Is This Level For?
Level III is for anyone who has done Level II for at least a month and who is very comfortable with the double moves.

Circuit Works
1. Since you've now built up a solid base of strength and endurance, shoot for 45–60 seconds per move, starting with 45 seconds and working your way up to 60.
2. Rest no more than 30 seconds between moves to improve recovery and burn tons of calories.
3. Go through each routine twice during the first week; go through each routine three times for Weeks 2–4.

Circuit Math
   10 moves @ 60 seconds each
+ 30 seconds rest in between moves
= 15 minutes each circuit (once through)

Which Weights?
Just as in previous levels, you might want to go through each routine once without weights to get used to the movements, since they take a bit of practice. Once you're familiar with them, begin with a slightly lighter weight than you were using in Level II and build up to heavier weights as you improve.

Cardio Rx
No more excuses: Do 45–60 minutes of solid cardio for your workouts this month!

Good Level III Cardio Ideas:
• jogging or running outside
• elliptical trainer with arms on an incline
• hill or stair jogging/running
• treadmill walking on an incline (6–10 percent)
• Stepmill or Stairmaster
• outdoor biking or advanced Spinning classes
• in-line skating

NOTABLE NOTES

As in Level II, you'll notice the basic movements used in each Level III move listed next to the move name. If you forget the form for a particular move, refer back to Level I for a refresher.

You'll notice that many of your Lower Body/Cardio moves this month are "plyometric," meaning you'll be catching some air! Pace yourself during these moves, as they are more difficult and require more energy. Also remember to land with your knees soft (slightly bent) to avoid injury.

Butt-Bi-Row (Biceps Curl / Upright Row / Glute Raise)

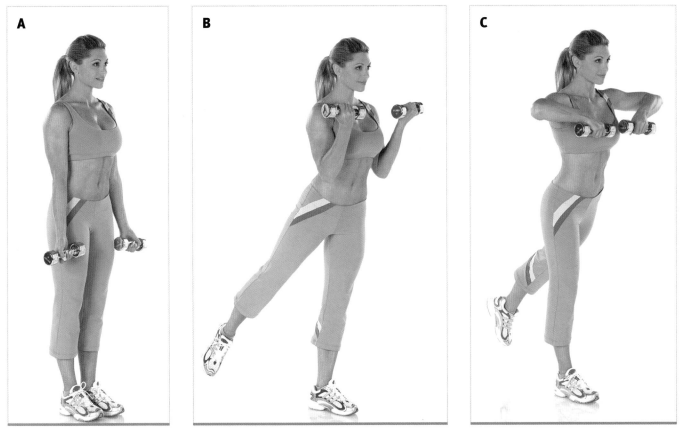

A. Stand with your feet together and your knees slightly bent, and hold a pair of dumbbells in front of your thighs, palms facing up.

B. Lift the weights in a biceps curl, simultaneously lifting your right leg straight behind you without arching your back (this is a glute raise).

C. Return your right leg to the start and lower the dumbbells (A). Turn your palms to face your thighs and lift the dumbbells up toward your chin in an upright row, simultaneously doing a glute raise with your left leg. Return the leg and dumbbells to the start. Repeat, alternating sides.

Balancing Biceps (Single Leg Squat / Biceps Curl)

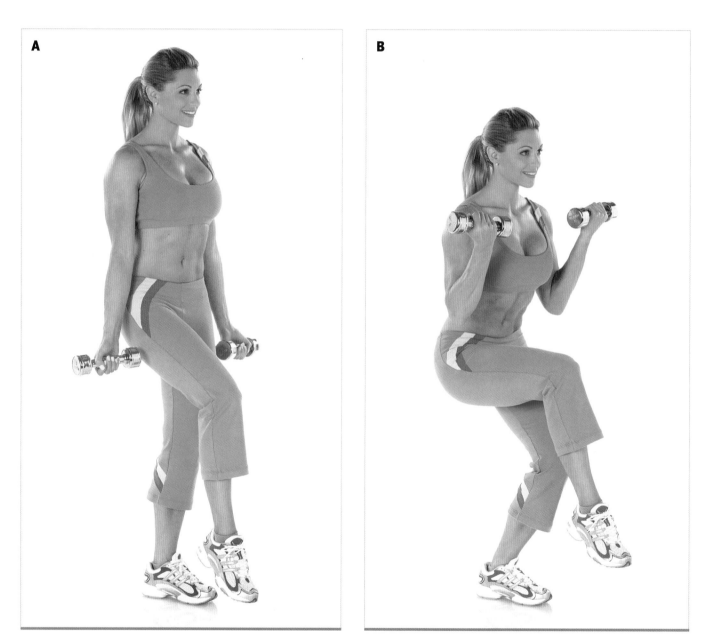

A **B**

A. Stand with your feet and knees together and hold a pair of dumbbells in front of your thighs, palms facing away from you. Shift your weight to your left side and lift your right foot off the floor, either curling it behind you or lifting it to the front of your body.

B. Squat toward the floor on your standing leg, simultaneously doing a biceps curl with your weights. Stand back up to the start and lower the dumbbells (A). Repeat, alternating legs every ten repetitions.

Supergirl Hamstring Curl
(Glute Raise / Overhead Shoulder Press / Hamstring Curl / Overhead Triceps Extension)

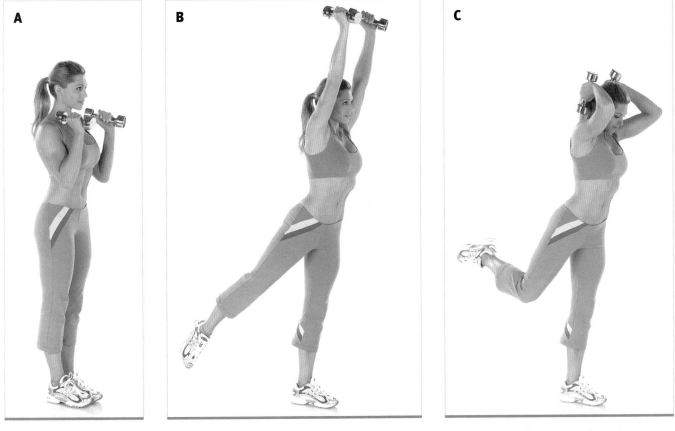

A. Stand with your feet together, and hold a pair of dumbbells by your shoulders, elbows down.

B. Simultaneously press the dumbbells up in an overhead shoulder press while lifting your right leg straight behind you in a glute raise.

C. Bend your elbows and drop the weights behind your head in a triceps extension while simultaneously bending your right knee to curl your heel toward your buttocks (this is a hamstring curl). Straighten your leg and your arms (B), and return to the start position (A). Repeat, alternating legs.

Side Lunge 'n' Lift 'n' Lift (Side Lunge / Floor Punch /Front Shoulder Raise / Glute Raise)

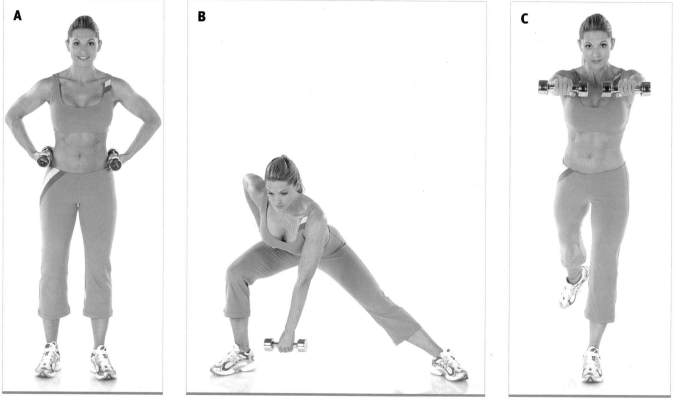

A. Stand with your feet hip-width apart, and rest your dumbbells on your hips, elbows out.

B. Do a side lunge to the right, simultaneously punching your left dumbbell down toward the floor.

C. Return to standing (A), and do a front shoulder raise with both arms while simultaneously doing a glute raise with your right leg. Repeat, alternating sides.

Kung Fu Reverse Lunge

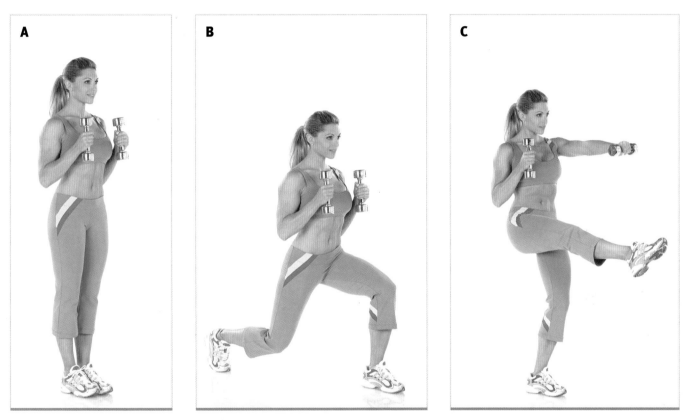

A. Stand with your feet together and hold a pair of dumbbells at shoulder height.

B. Take a large step backward with your right foot in a reverse lunge.

C. When your left thigh is parallel to the floor, push off your right foot, straightening your left leg. Bring your right leg through, kicking it to the front of your body at hip height. Simultaneously extend your left hand forward in a cross punch. Step back through to the rear with your right leg (B) and repeat. Alternate sides, doing 10 repetitions with each leg.

Super Squat (Squat / Overhead Shoulder Press / Close Squat / 90-Degree Chest Fly)

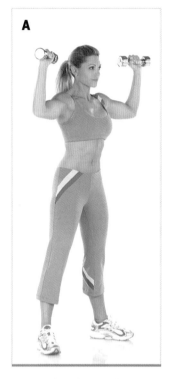

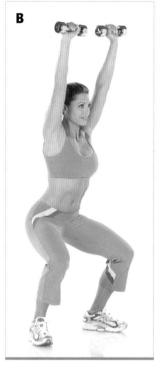

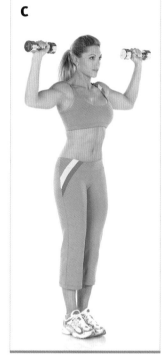

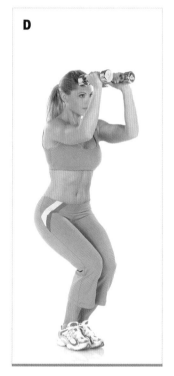

A. Stand with your feet hip-width apart and hold a pair dumbbells at ear level, wrists stacked over elbows, palms facing forward.

B. Do a slow basic squat, simultaneously pressing the weights straight up in an overhead shoulder press.

C. As you return to standing, simultaneously step your feet together and lower the weights back to ear level.

D. Do a slow close squat, simultaneously bringing your elbows together in front of your head in a 90-degree chest fly. Return to standing and open your arms (C) to complete one repetition.

Balancing Booty Burner (Right)
(Reverse Lunge—Left / Glute Raise and Balance / Rear Shoulder Fly)

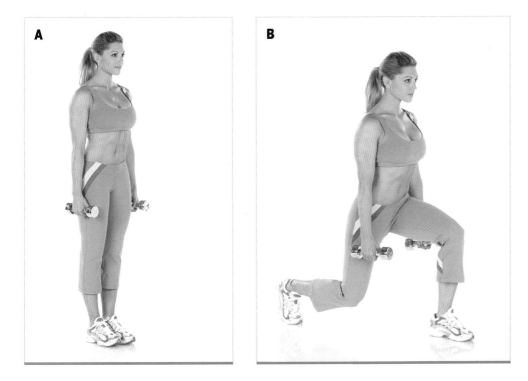

A. Stand with your feet together and hold a pair of dumbbells at your sides.

B. Do a reverse lunge with your right leg.

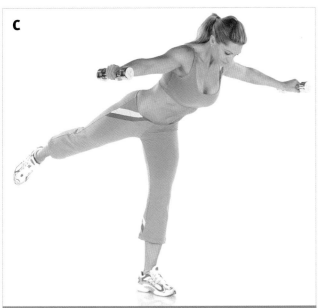

C. Straighten your legs, then pick your right foot up off the ground and lift it behind you, simultaneously tipping forward with your upper body until your torso is almost parallel to the floor. Balance here as you do a rear shoulder fly (as shown). Place your right foot back on the floor behind you, lower into another lunge (B), and repeat.

Balancing Booty Burner (Left) (Reverse Lunge—Right / Glute Raise /Bent-Over Row)

A. Stand with your feet together and hold a pair of dumbbells at your sides.

B. Do a reverse lunge with your left leg.

C. Straighten your legs, then pick your left foot up off the ground and lift it behind you, simultaneously tipping forward with your upper body until your torso is nearly parallel to the floor. Balance here as you do a bent-over row (as shown). Place your left foot back on the floor, lower into another lunge (B), and repeat.

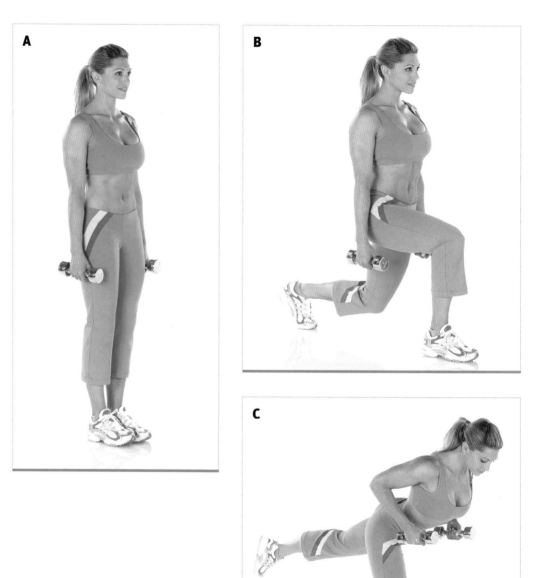

Ballet Super-Squat Combo (Ballet Squat / Calf Raise / Upright Row)

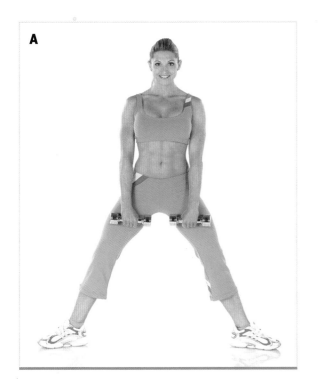

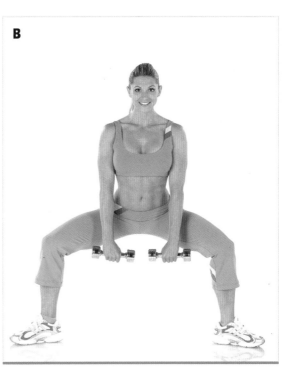

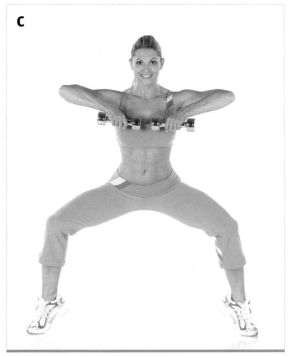

A. Stand with your feet double hip–width apart and turn your legs out from the hips so your knees and toes are pointing on the diagonal. Hold a pair of dumbbells in front of your body, palms facing your thighs.

B. Do a slow ballet squat, stopping when your thighs are parallel to the floor.

C. Hold here and lift your heels off the floor in a calf raise, simultaneously lifting the dumbbells toward your chin in an upright row. Lower the weights and your heels and stand back up to the start.

Steam Engine

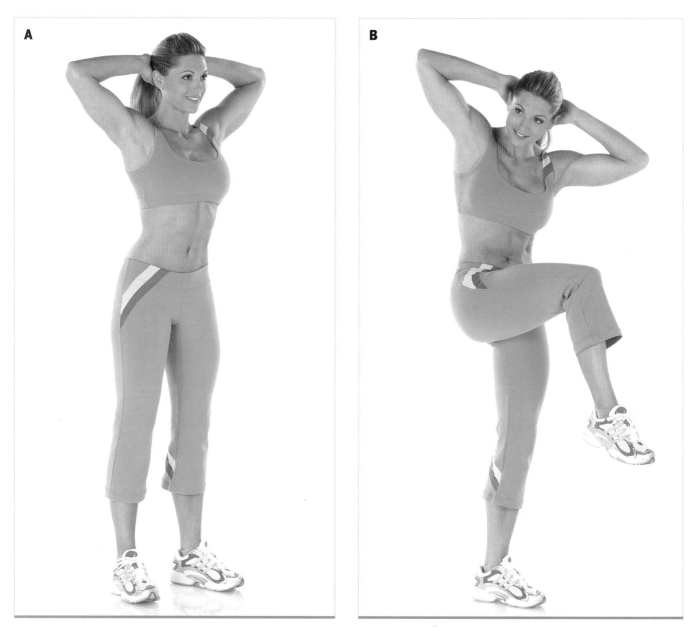

A. Stand with your feet hip-width apart and place your hands behind your head, elbows pointing out from your ears.

B. Bring one knee up in front of your body to hip height, and twist with your upper body, reaching your opposite elbow toward the lifted knee. Alternate sides rhythmically, starting off slowly and increasing your speed as your time runs out.

Low Flow (Triceps Kickback / Step Out / Punch)

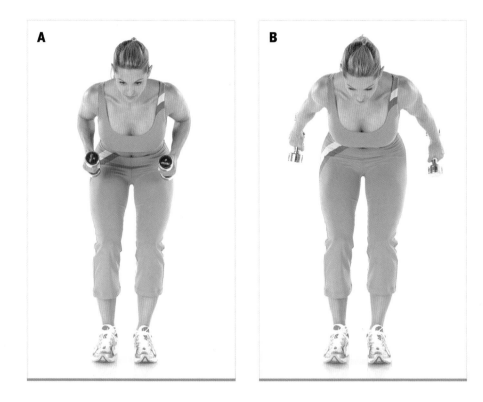

A. Stand with your feet hip-width apart and bend forward from your waist until your torso is almost parallel to the floor. Bend your arms and pin your elbows to your sides.

B. Do a slow repetition of a triceps extension.

C. Now turn and punch your right hand across your body to the left at shoulder height while extending your right leg to the side. Return to the start (A), do another triceps extension (B), then punch and lunge on the opposite side. Repeat in a rhythmic pattern, staying as low as possible throughout the move.

Seesaw (Deadlift / Bent-Over Row / Rear Shoulder Fly)

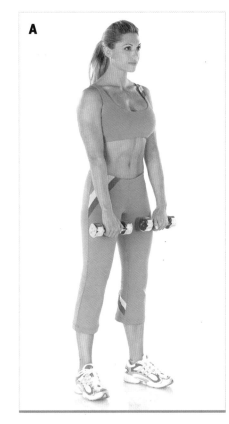

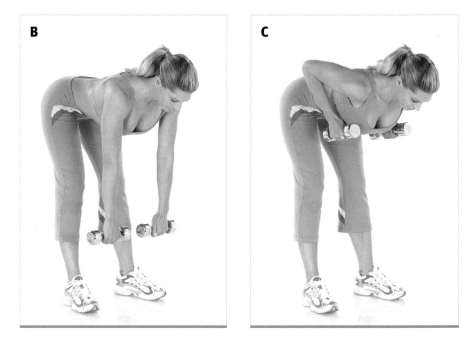

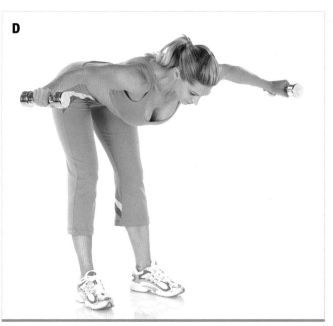

A. Stand with your feet and knees shoulder-width apart and hold a pair of dumbbells in front of your thighs.

B. Slowly bend forward from the waist until your torso is almost parallel to the floor, keeping your legs straight and your back flat (this is a deadlift position). Allow your arms to hang down from your shoulders.

C. Lift the weights toward your chest in a bent-over row. Extend your arms (B), stand slowly back to the start (A), and immediately lower once more into the deadlift position (B).

D. Hold here and raise your arms up and out to your sides in a rear shoulder fly. Return your arms to the start (B), and stand up once more (A) to complete one repetition.

Split-Hand Push-up

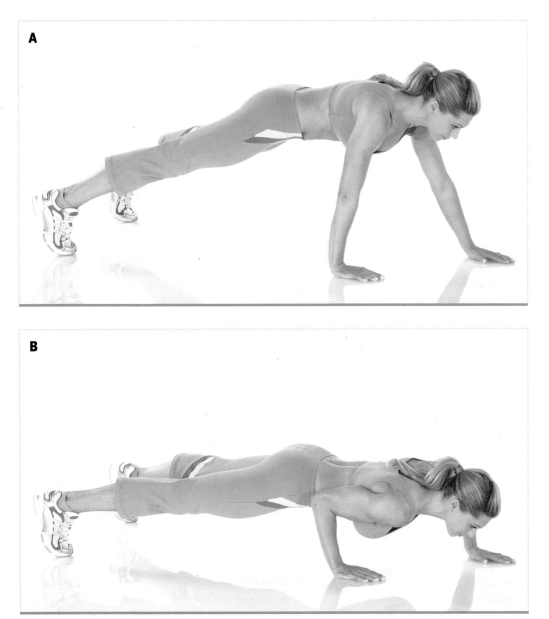

A. Get in a push-up position on the floor and spread your feet about shoulder-width apart. Place your left hand slightly in front of your shoulder on the floor and your right hand closer to your body by your rib cage.

B. Bend your elbows and lower your torso toward the floor, keeping your abs tight and your hips lifted. Do 10 repetitions in this position, then switch your hands so your left hand is close to your body and your right hand is in front. Alternate sides until your time runs out.

Advanced Superman

A. Lie facedown on the floor with your legs together and your arms stretched overhead along the floor.

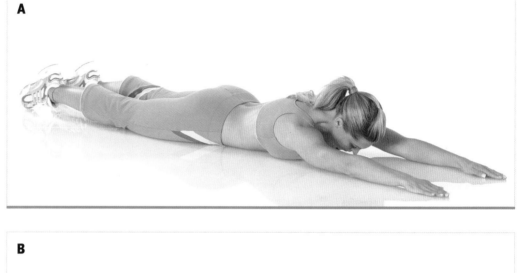

B. Raise all four limbs off the floor simultaneously and hold for two breaths. Slowly lower to the start and repeat right away.

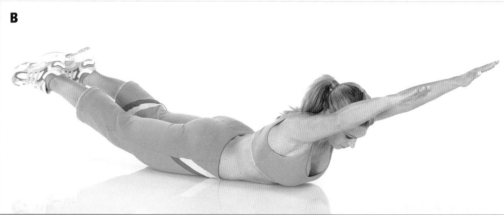

Plank Plus

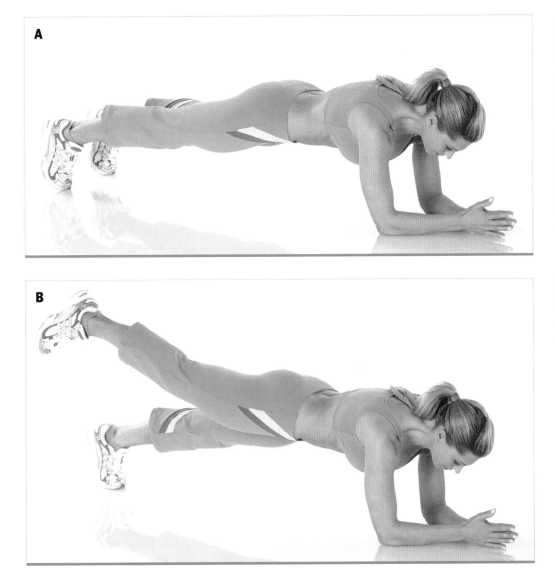

A. Lie facedown on the floor with your legs extended behind you and your toes turned under, and line your elbows up underneath your shoulders, pressing your palms together underneath your chin. Lift your torso, hips, and thighs off the ground into a plank position.

B. Hold this position and lift your right leg off the floor without letting your hips tilt or your butt sag. Hold for two breaths, then lower your right leg and lift your left leg, holding for two breaths. Continue, alternating sides.

Bridge Bonus

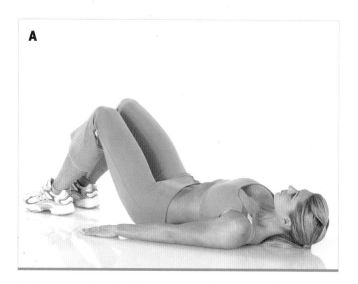

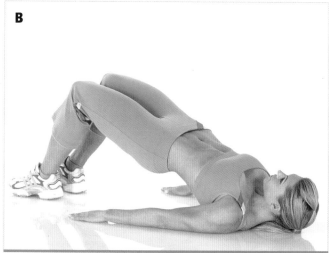

A. Lie on your back with your arms along your sides, your knees bent, and your feet flat on the floor.

B. Squeeze your glutes and hamstrings to lift your hips into the air in a bridge position.

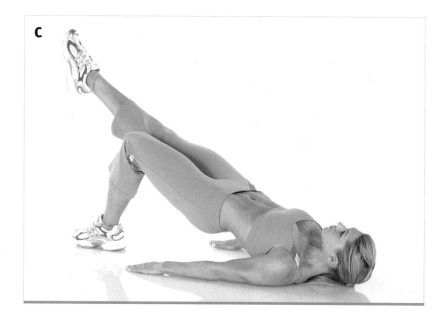

C. Hold your body up with your left leg as you straighten your right leg and hold it in the air. Hold for two breaths, then lower your left leg and extend your right leg. Repeat, alternating sides, keeping your hips lifted in the bridge position throughout.

Reach-for-the-Sky Crunch

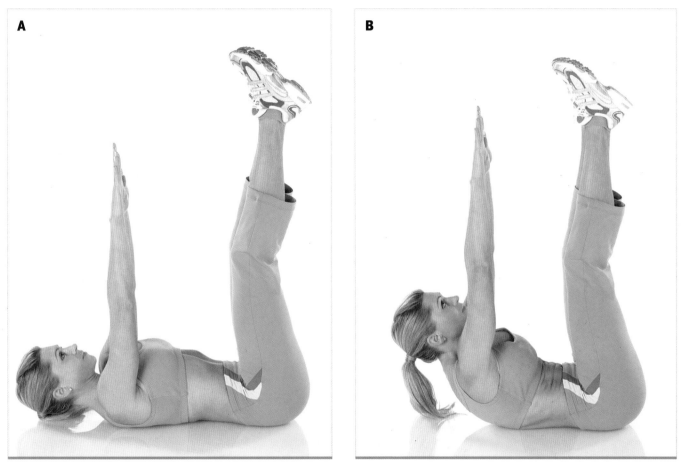

A. Lie on your back with your legs straight and lifted over your hips and your arms extended straight up, your fingers pointing toward the ceiling.

B. Reach with straight arms toward your toes, lifting your head, shoulders, and upper back off the floor. Lower back to the start and repeat right away.

Punch Crunch

A. Lie on your back with your knees bent and lifted above your hips. Make fists with your hands and bring them to your shoulders.

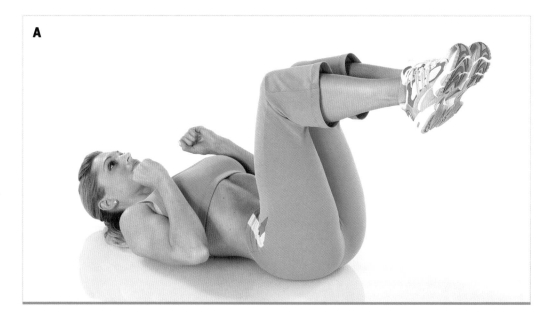

B. Lift your head, shoulders, and upper back off the floor, simultaneously twisting to the right and punching across your body with your left hand. Lower to the start and repeat, alternating sides.

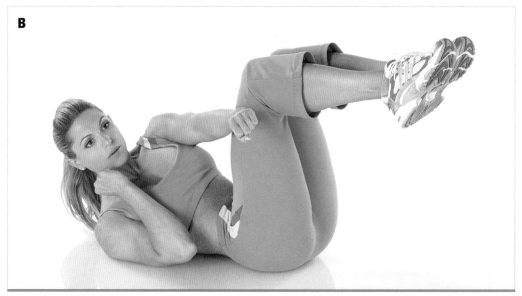

Donkey Kick Bonus

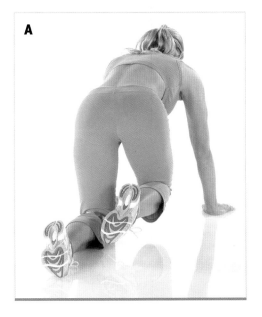

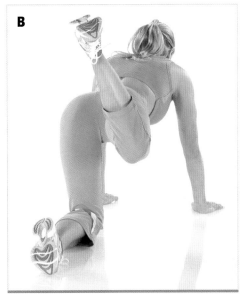

A. Get on all fours with your hands directly underneath your shoulders and your knees directly underneath your hips, one knee lifted slightly off the floor.

B. Press your right leg behind you, pushing your heel toward the ceiling, with your knee bent and your foot flexed in a donkey kick.

C. As you lower your right leg back toward the floor, cross it behind your left leg. Lift it up toward the ceiling once more, then return it to the floor. Repeat, alternating sides.

Straight-Leg Donkey Kick Bonus

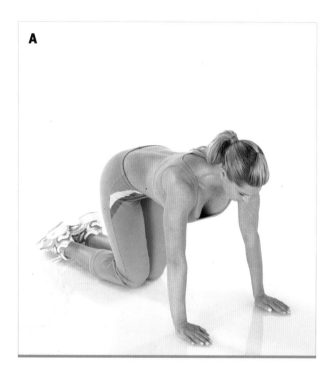

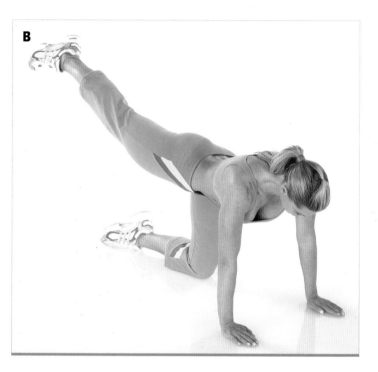

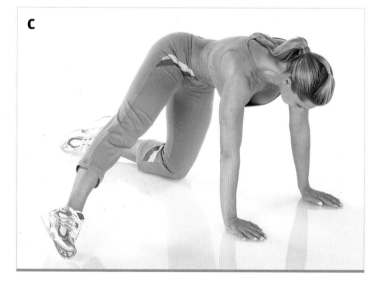

A. Get on all fours with your hands directly underneath your shoulders and your knees directly underneath your hips.

B. Extend one leg and lift it toward the ceiling in a straight-leg glute raise.

C. Keep your leg elevated and slowly open it to the side of your body, drawing an arc though the air with your toe parallel to the floor. Bring your leg back behind you (B), and lower it back to the floor (A). Repeat, alternating sides.

Windmill Plank (Plank / Side Plank)

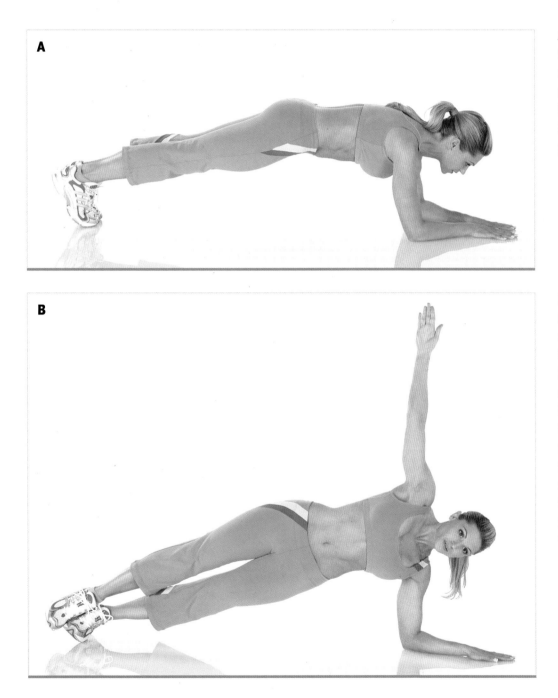

A. Start in a plank position with your elbows directly underneath your shoulders, your palms flat on the floor, and your legs extended behind you.

B. Open your body to the side and stack your feet and hips in a side plank, balancing on your left forearm. Extend your right arm toward the ceiling in line with your shoulders. Hold for two breaths, then place your right forearm back on the floor, return momentarily to the plank position, then repeat the side plank on the left. Alternate sides.

Mountain Climber

A. Start in a push-up position with your legs together and your hands underneath your shoulders.

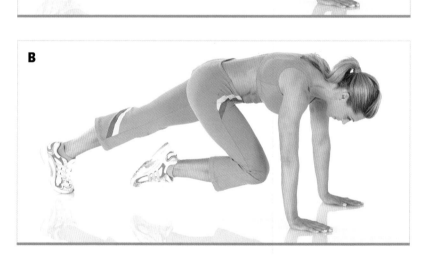

B. Bring one knee in toward your chest, keeping your butt low and your hips square, and hold for one breath.

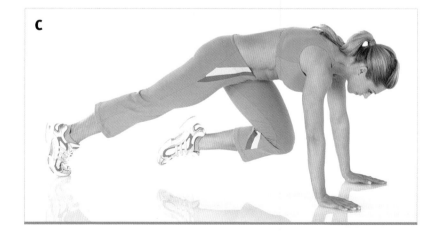

C. Return to the start. Repeat, alternating sides. **Note:** Do this move slowly at first; then, as you improve, do it faster and faster until you can "run" in place.

Full Power Lunge

A. Stand with your feet together and your arms at your sides.

B. Jump your feet apart, landing in a deep lunge with your right foot forward and your left foot back.

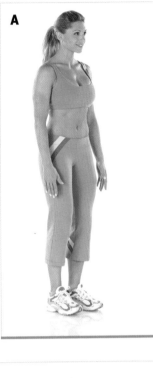

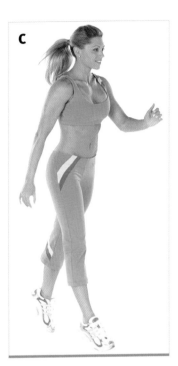

C. Immediately spring back into the air, switching feet.

D. Land with your left foot forward and your right foot back. Repeat steps B, C, and D, alternating sides rhythmically.

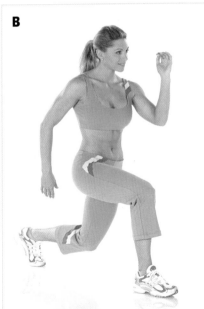

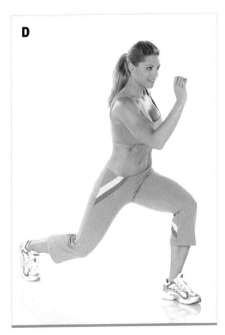

Hop Around the Clock

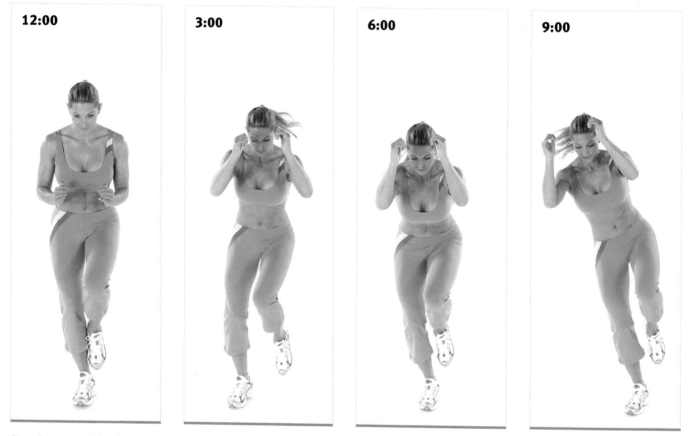

12:00 | **3:00** | **6:00** | **9:00**

Stand on you right foot with your knee slightly bent, and imagine you're standing in the middle of a giant clock face. Hop to the 12 (directly in front of you), then back to the center. Then hop to the 3 (to your right) and back to the

center. Continue this pattern for the 6 (behind you) and the 9 (to your left). Repeat, circling clockwise, then switch to your left foot. Alternate sides until your time runs out.

High-Knee Run

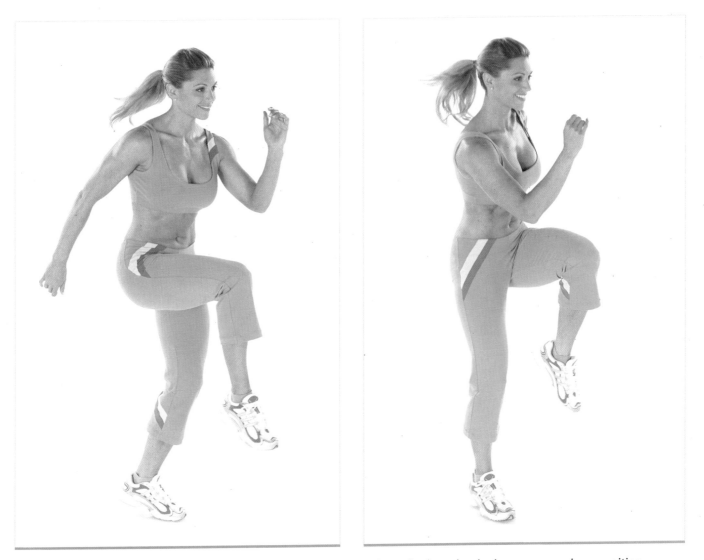

Run in place, bringing your knees as high as you can to the front of your body and swinging your arms in opposition.

Plyo Squat

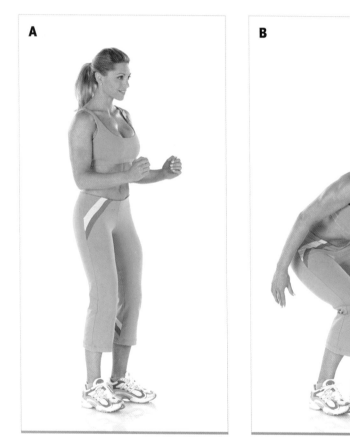

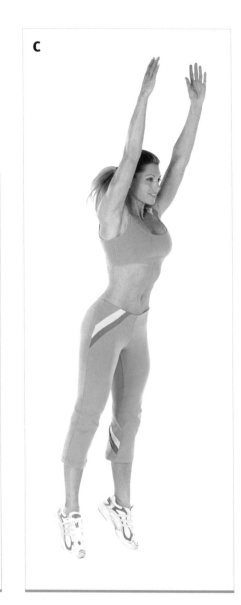

A. Stand with your feet hip-width apart and parallel, your arms at your sides with your elbows bent.

B. Lower into a basic squat, bringing your arms down by your sides.

C. When your thighs are almost parallel to the floor, jump off the ground, lifting your arms into the air to help you gain elevation. Land with your knees soft, and immediately lower into the next squat and jump. Repeat rhythmically.

Mogul Jump

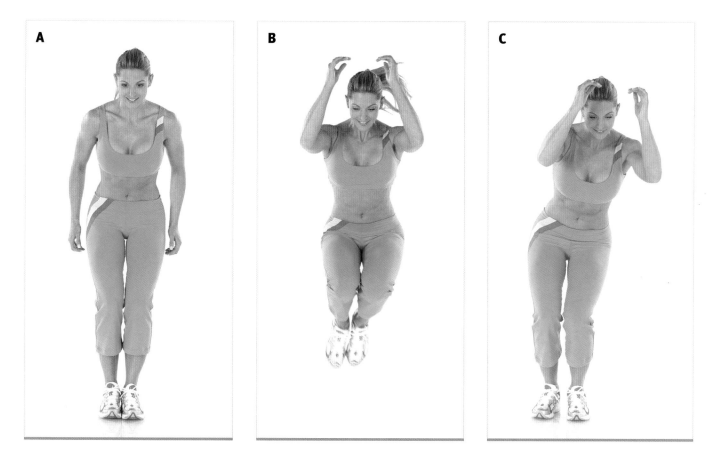

A. With your feet and knees together, jump from side to side over an imaginary snow mogul.

B. Lift your knees and tuck your feet underneath you to get as much air as possible!

C. Use your arms to help you leap into the air, and remember to land with soft knees.

Tuck Jack

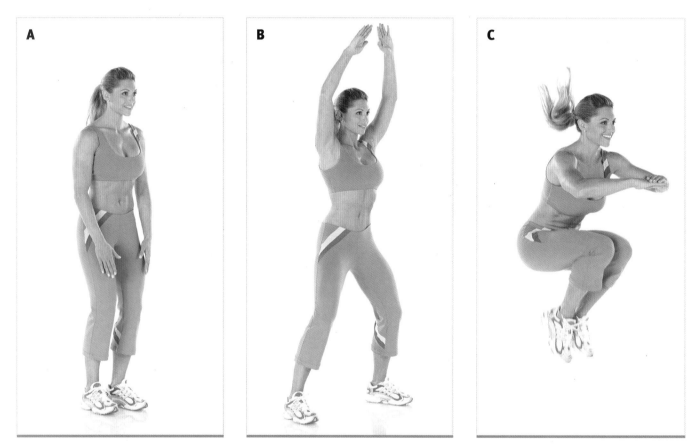

A. Stand with your feet and knees together and your arms at your sides.

B. Lightly jump your feet apart into a wide stance and raise your arms completely overhead.

C. Immediately jump back to the start (A) and then leap straight up into the air, bringing your knees toward your chest and tucking your feet underneath you. Land with soft knees to complete one repetition. Repeat in a rhythmic pattern.

Super Speed Skate

A. Stand with your feet together and your arms at your sides. Bend forward from the waist, keeping your back flat, and bend your knees.

B. Take a big leap to the right side with your right leg, staying low. Touch the floor by your right foot with your left hand as you bring your left foot behind and across your right leg.

C. Immediately push off your right foot and leap to the left side, touching the floor with your right hand. Alternate sides rhythmically, repeating steps B and C.

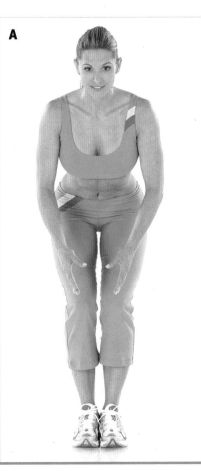

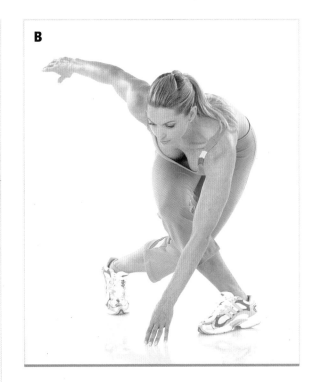

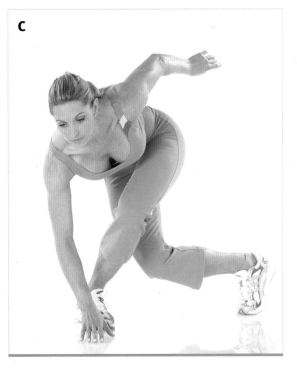

Pop Squat

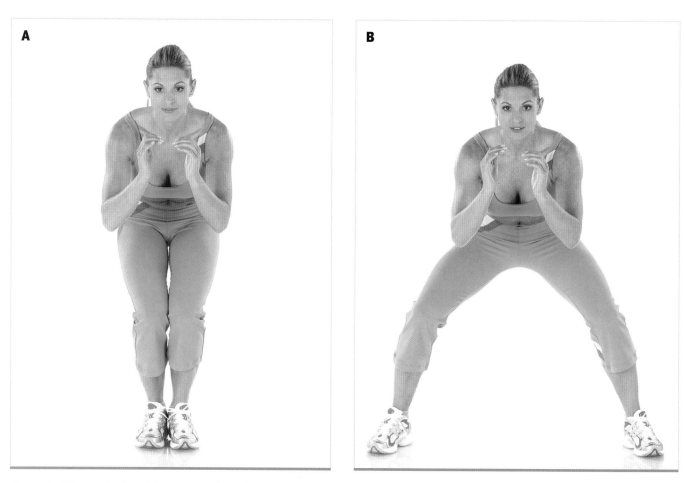

A. Start with your feet and knees together, then squat down halfway into a close squat.

B. From here, jump your feet apart into a wide basic squat, then right back together in a close squat (A). Repeat rhythmically, staying low in this half-squat position throughout the move!

Power Burpee

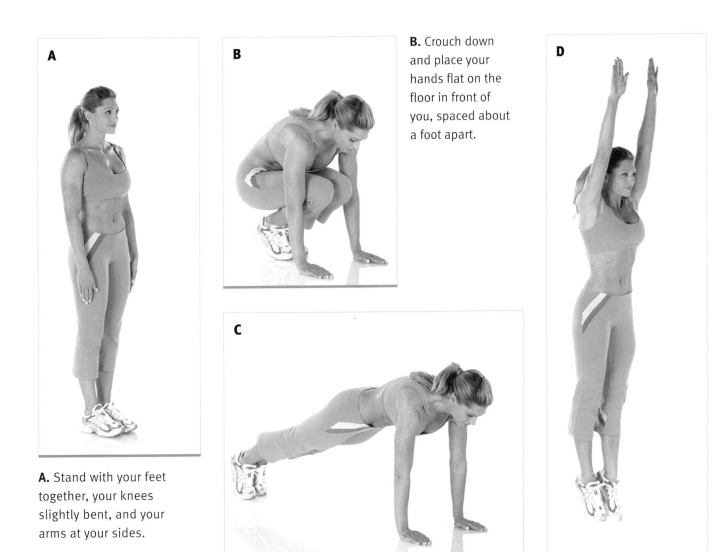

A. Stand with your feet together, your knees slightly bent, and your arms at your sides.

B. Crouch down and place your hands flat on the floor in front of you, spaced about a foot apart.

C. Hop both feet behind you into a push-up position.

D. Immediately hop both feet back underneath your hips into a crouch position (B), then jump into the air from the crouch, raising your arms overhead. Land with your knees soft and repeat sequence right away.

Level III Suggested Schedule

WEEK	MONDAY	TUESDAY	WEDNESDAY	THURSDAY	FRIDAY	SATURDAY	SUNDAY
1	Circuit 1	Lower Body/ Cardio	Circuit 2 and Cardio (45–50 minutes)	Rest	Lower Body/Cardio and Trouble Spots	Either Circuit 1 or Circuit 2	Rest
2	Circuit 1	Lower Body/ Cardio	Circuit 2 and Cardio (45–50 minutes)	Rest	Lower Body/Cardio and Trouble Spots	Either Circuit 1 or Circuit 2	Rest
3	Circuit 1 and Trouble Spots	Lower Body/ Cardio	Circuit 2 and Cardio (50–60 minutes)	Rest	Lower Body/Cardio and Trouble Spots	Either Circuit 1 or Circuit 2	Rest
4	Circuit 1 and Trouble Spots	Lower Body/ Cardio	Circuit 2 and Cardio (50–60 minutes)	Rest	Lower Body/Cardio and Trouble Spots	Either Circuit 1 or Circuit 2	Rest

Week 1: Do each circuit twice.

Week 2: Do each circuit twice or 3 times.

Week 3: Do each circuit 3 times.

Week 4: Do each circuit 3 times.

CIRCUIT 1
1. Butt-Bi-Row
2. Full Power Lunge
3. Supergirl Hamstring Curl
4. Plyo Squat
5. Side Lunge 'n' Lift 'n' Lift
6. Kung Fu Reverse Lunge
7. Seesaw
8. Mogul Jump
9. Super Squat
10. Tuck Jack

CIRCUIT 2
1. Balancing Biceps
2. Super Speed Skate
3. Low Flow
4. Power Burpee
5. Balancing Booty Burner (Left)
6. Ballet Super-Squat Combo
7. Balancing Booty Burner (Right)
8. Pop Squat
9. Steam Engine
10. High-Knee Run

LOWER BODY/CARDIO
1. High-Knee Run
2. Mogul Jump
3. Pop Squat
4. Side Lunge 'n' Lift 'n' Lift
5. Plyo Squat
6. Full Power Lunge
7. Hop Around the Clock
8. Super Speed Skate
9. Power Burpee
10. Tuck Jack

TROUBLE SPOTS WORKOUT
1. Split-Hand Push-up
2. Advanced Superman
3. Plank Plus
4. Donkey Kick Bonus
5. Windmill Plank
6. Mountain Climbers
7. Straight-Leg Donkey Kick Bonus
8. Bridge Bonus
9. Reach-for-the-Sky Crunch
10. Punch Crunch

STRETCHING

Have you ever watched a baby effortlessly grab her toes and stick them in her mouth? Once upon a time we were all that flexible, and while you may not be able to chew your toenails again (or want to, for that matter!), you can certainly improve your flexibility with regular training.

Ideally, you should dedicate 10–20 minutes every day to flexibility training to improve your body's range of motion, decrease muscle soreness and stiffness, and help alleviate chronic back, neck, and shoulder pain. I recommend doing your flexibility work after your workouts, when your muscles are warm and supple, not only as a good stretch but also as an effective cool-down.

Some of these moves might be challenging at first, but don't be discouraged! Make it one of your goals to master them in time.

Points of Focus
• holding each stretch for 15–30 seconds
• breathing deeply
• relaxing and releasing tension
• pushing yourself to the point of slight discomfort, but not to the point of pain
• slowly increasing range of motion with each session

Standing Calf Stretch

Muscles stretched: Calves

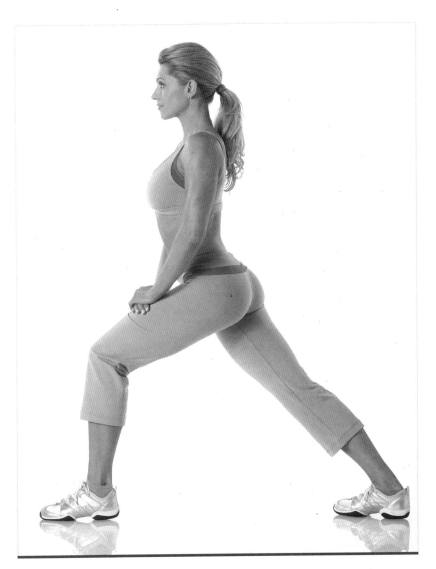

Stand with your feet apart in a wide lunge stance, with your back knee straight and your front knee slightly bent. Press your rear heel toward the floor and hold. For a slightly different stretch, keep your heel down, and slowly bend and straighten your rear knee.

Standing Quad Stretch

Muscles stretched: Quadriceps

Stand with your feet hip-width apart, and bend your left knee to bring your left heel up toward your buttocks. Grab your left foot with your left hand and hold it, tucking your tailbone slightly underneath you. Make sure your knee is pointing toward the floor and that you're not tipping to one side or the other. If you have trouble with balance, place one hand on a chair or sturdy object. Repeat on your right side.

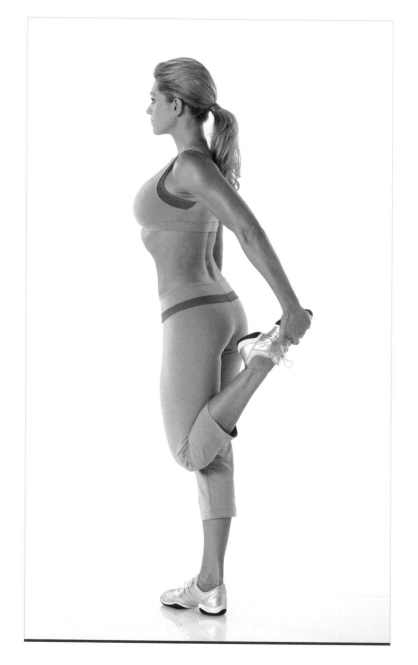

Standing Side Stretch

Muscles stretched: Sides, shoulders, obliques, back, hips

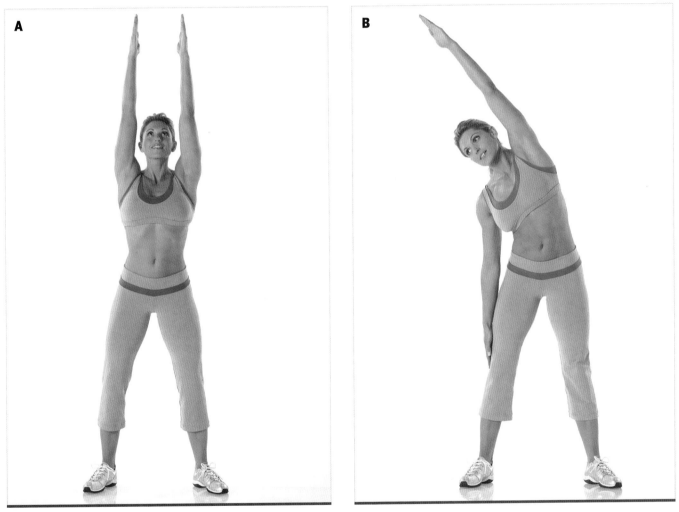

A. Stand with your feet double hip–width apart and your knees slightly bent, and reach both arms overhead, elbows by your ears.

B. Slowly drop over to the right side, lowering your right arm to support your weight along your right leg while reaching up and over your head with your left arm. Keep your hips square and your feet flat on the floor. Repeat on the left side by reaching into the air with your right hand and supporting your weight with your left.

Standing Torso Hang

Muscles stretched: Hamstrings, lower back, shoulders, neck

Stand with your feet double hip–width apart and your knees slightly bent. Slowly roll your torso down toward the floor and allow your upper body to hang freely. You can let your arms hang down from your shoulders or cross them over each other (as shown). Focus on relaxing your neck, hamstrings, and back. For an extra stretch, turn your head slowly from side to side as you hang.

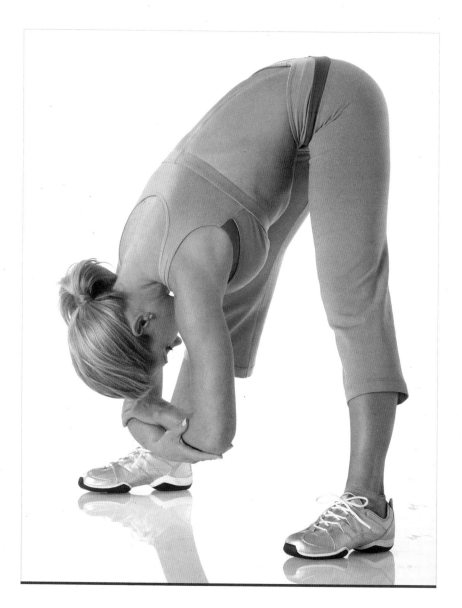

Shoulder Stretch

Muscles stretched: Rear and lateral deltoids

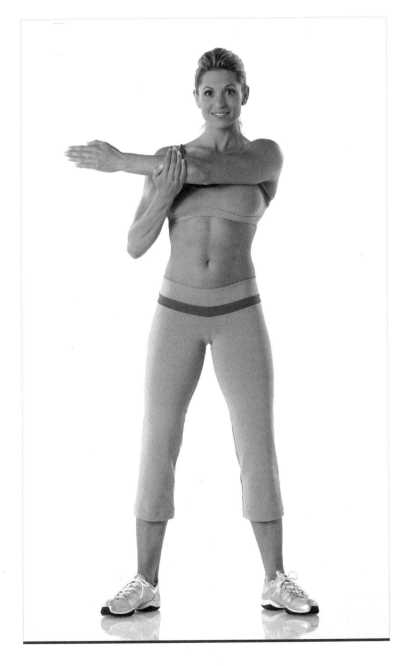

Bring your left arm across your body at chest height and grab your left forearm with your right hand. Actively press your left shoulder down—don't allow it to shrug up by your ear—as you stretch your arm across your body. For a deeper stretch, tilt your head away from your left shoulder. Repeat on the other side.

Triceps Stretch

Muscles stretched: Triceps, sides

Bring your left arm straight up by your ear, and bend your elbow so your hand drops behind your head and touches your right shoulder. With your right hand, reach over your head to clasp your left elbow, pulling your left arm toward your right side behind your head. Repeat on the other side.

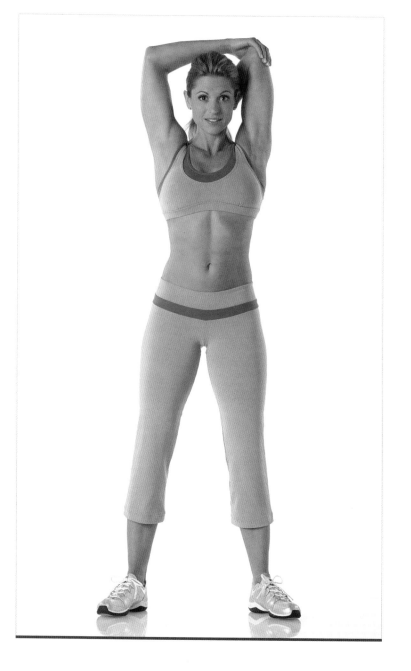

Chest Stretch

Muscles stretched: Chest, front deltoids, biceps, neck

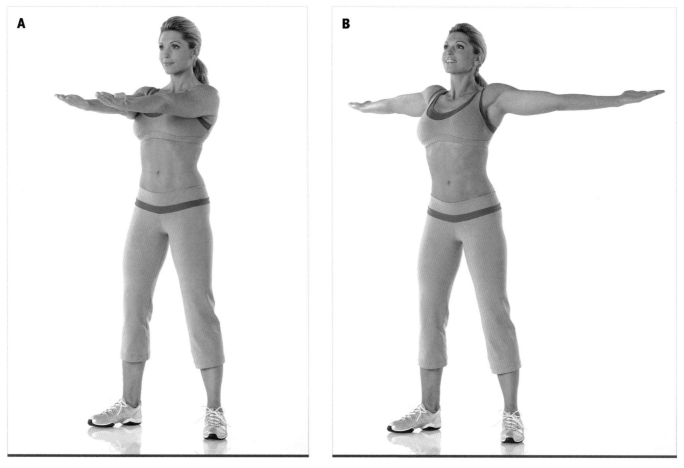

A. Stand with your feet double hip–width apart and raise both arms to shoulder height in front of your body, palms up.

B. Exhale and open your arms out and back as wide as you can, thumbs pointing behind you. Lift your chest up slightly and tilt your chin toward the ceiling. Rotate your arms (palms up/palms down) in this open position.

Crouching Stretch

Muscles stretched: Inner thighs, hips, glutes

Stand with your feet double hip–width apart, your toes and knees turned out slightly on the diagonal, and squat down until your thighs are parallel to the floor. Your knees should be over your ankles. Place your elbows inside your thighs and press outward, stretching your thighs open. Hold here and breathe. You can also rock back and forth slightly to increase the stretch.

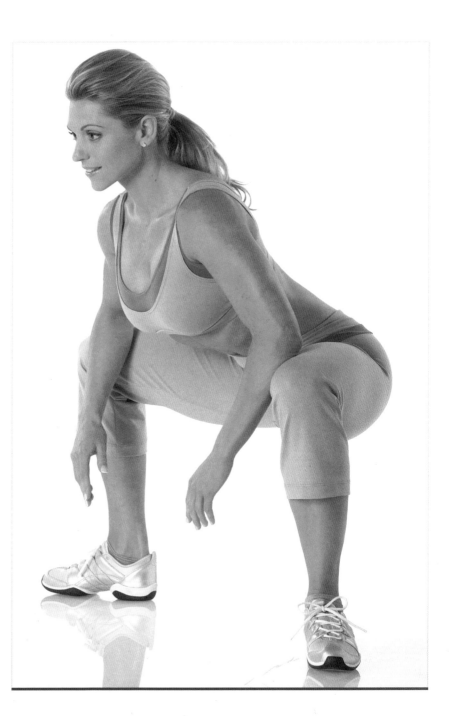

Runner's Lunge

Muscles stretched: Hip flexors, inner thighs, glutes

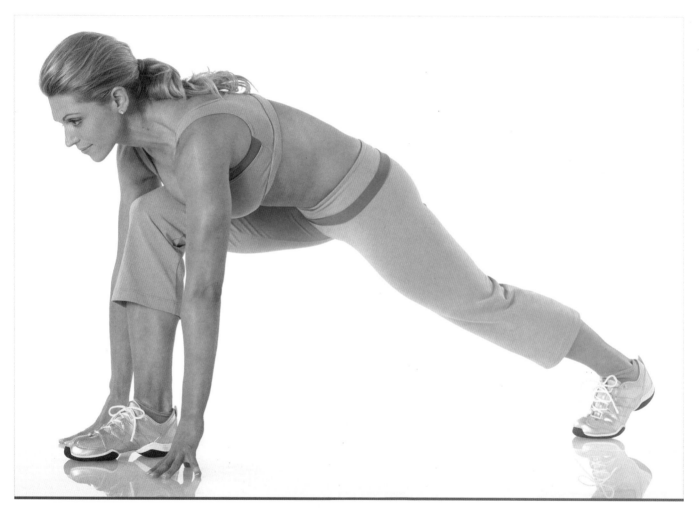

Stand in a really wide lunge with your right foot forward. Place your hands on either side of your right foot and fold your upper body over your right thigh. Keep your right knee over your toes and your left leg straight. Hold and breathe, feeling the stretch through the front of your left hip. Repeat on the other side.

Neck Stretch

Muscles stretched: Neck, trapezius

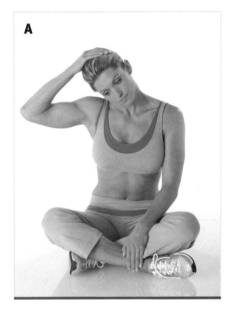

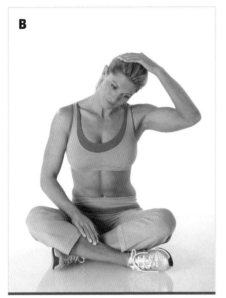

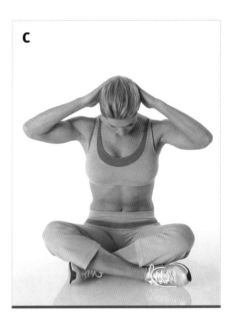

A. Sit cross-legged on the floor with your shoulders relaxed, and drop your right ear to your right shoulder. Place your right hand on the left side of your head and—without pulling—let the weight of your arm gently stretch your neck for 10–15 seconds.

B. Repeat on the left side.

C. Then drop your chin to your chest, place both hands behind your head, hold, and stretch. For an additional tension-relieving stretch, slowly roll your head in a large semicircle to the front, dropping your left ear to your left shoulder, then roll your head around to the right side. Repeat, alternating sides.

Cat/Dog

Muscles stretched: Back, chest, hip flexors, glutes, shoulders

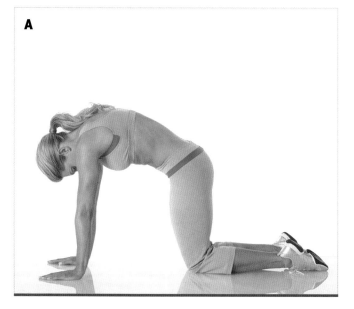

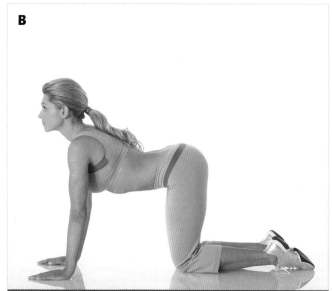

A. Get on all fours with your hands directly underneath your shoulders and your knees directly underneath your hips. Take a big breath in and round your back up like a Halloween cat, dropping your head and tucking your tailbone under.

B. Exhale and reverse the motion, arching your back and lifting your chin toward the ceiling and your tailbone toward the sky. Repeat, alternating positions slowly in time with your breathing.

Single-Leg Hamstring Stretch

Muscles stretched: Hamstrings, lower back, upper back, shoulders

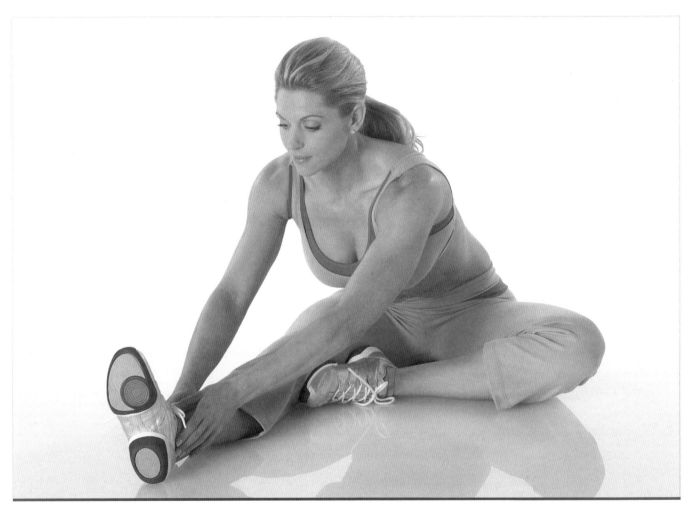

Sit on the floor with your right leg extended straight out from the hip and your foot flexed. Bend your left knee and place the sole of your left shoe alongside your right knee, allowing your left knee to fall outward from the hip. Reach with both hands toward your right foot and hold. Repeat on the other side.

Seated Butterfly Stretch

Muscles stretched: Inner thigh, hips, back, shoulders

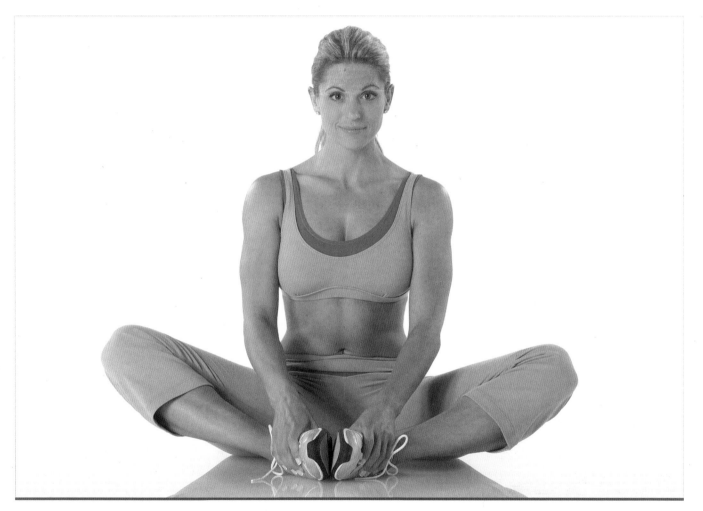

Sit on the floor and place the soles of your feet together, allowing your knees to fall away from each other. Hold your feet with both hands and, with a flat back, lean forward over your legs and hold.

Lying Glute Stretch

Muscles stretched: Glutes, hips

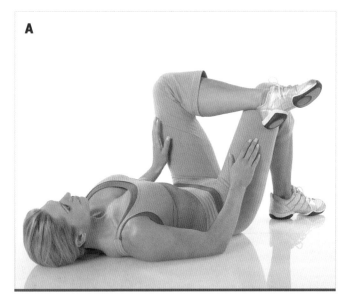

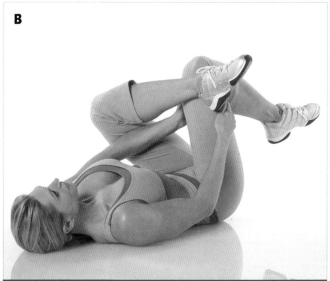

A. Lie on your back with your knees bent and your feet flat on the floor. Lift your left leg, bend your left knee, and place your left ankle across your right thigh. If this is enough of a stretch for you, hold this position and breathe.

B. If you need more of a challenge, lift both legs off the floor and pull them in toward your chest, holding your right thigh with both hands. Repeat on the other side.

Lying Spinal Twist

Muscles stretched: Back, hips, shoulders, neck

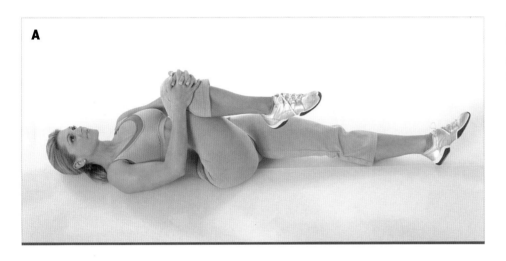

A. Lie on the floor with your legs together. Bend your right knee and bring it in to your chest, holding it with both hands.

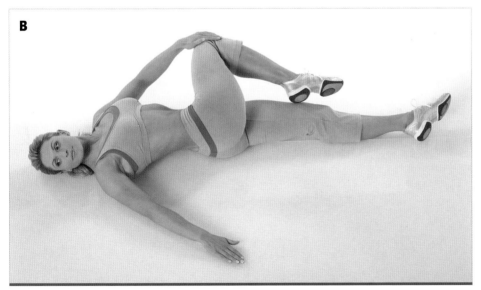

B. Then pull your knee across your body to the left side, extending your right arm along the floor and turning your head to the right. Use your left hand to pull your knee farther toward the floor with each breath, and focus on trying to get your right shoulder as close to the floor as possible. Repeat on the other side.

SAMPLE STRETCHING ROUTINE

Do these moves in the order suggested as a good cool-down after a workout as well as a great stretching workout (24 moves @ 30 seconds per move = 12 minutes).

1. Standing Calf Stretch, Right Leg
2. Standing Calf Stretch, Left Leg
3. Standing Quad Stretch, Right Leg
4. Standing Quad Stretch, Left Leg
5. Standing Side Stretch, Right Side
6. Standing Side Stretch, Left Side
7. Chest Stretch
8. Shoulder Stretch, Right Side
9. Triceps Stretch, Right side
10. Shoulder Stretch, Left Side
11. Triceps Stretch, Left Side
12. Standing Torso Hang
13. Crouching Stretch
14. Runner's Lunge, Right Side
15. Runner's Lunge, Left Side
16. Single-Leg Hamstring Stretch, Right Side
17. Single-Leg Hamstring Stretch, Left Side
18. Seated Butterfly Stretch
19. Neck Stretch
20. Lying Glute Stretch, Right Side
21. Lying Spinal Twist, Right Side
22. Lying Glute Stretch, Left Side
23. Lying Spinal Twist, Left Side
24. Cat/Dog

CHAPTER 10

Injury Prevention

Injuries happen. You probably don't want to hear that, and I certainly don't want to scare you. But even the most dedicated and elite athletes experience injuries from time to time. Whether you're a beginning exerciser or an Ironman triathlete, it's important to understand injuries so you can better prevent them. My rule of thumb is always this: An ounce of prevention is better than four months of rehab!

The good news is you're already taking steps to stay healthy and injury free just by exercising! Resistance training, flexibility work, and cardio help strengthen bones, ligaments, and tendons, significantly lowering your risk for injury. So keep that up, and read this chapter carefully to prevent injury and enjoy exercise for years to come.

KINDS OF INJURIES

There are basically two kinds of exercise injuries: acute and overuse. Acute injuries are usually the result of a single, traumatic event such as a fall or an impact that causes damage to a joint or a muscle. These injuries are often accompanied by sharp pain, swelling, bruising, and loss of mobility in the injured part. Some examples of acute injuries are wrist fractures, ankle sprains, and shoulder dislocations.

Overuse injuries, on the other hand, are a bit harder to pin down, as they occur over time as the result of repetitive microtrauma to the tendons, bones, and joints. They typically start off as a small, nagging ache or pain and, if left untreated or ignored, can grow into a chronic, more serious condition. They can be the result of trying to do too much activity too soon, using poor workout technique, or muscle imbalances. Shin splints, tendonitis, bursitis, and stress fractures are examples of overuse injuries.

BURNING QUESTION

What is cross-training? Cross-training simply means doing a variety of different activities to use your muscles in different ways. If you always do the same kind of workout, you're more likely to experience overuse injuries from repetitive movements. For instance, a long-distance runner spends hours doing the same activity—running. For a runner to

Fun Fact
Men are 30 percent more likely to injure themselves than women!

reduce her risk for injury, she should cross-train with activities other than running, such as cycling, swimming, or resistance training, to use her muscles in different ways. The greater variety of activities you can do, the less your risk of injury will be.

RELATIVE REST, ICE, COMPRESSION, AND ELEVATION (RICE)

Many minor injuries can be treated by using RICE, an acronym for relative rest, ice, compression, and elevation. As soon as you think you've injured yourself—be it an acute or overuse incident—apply RICE, then, if necessary, contact your physician.

- **Relative Rest** In order to ensure proper healing, it's important to rest the injured area. For example, if you have an ankle sprain, you certainly shouldn't go out for a jog. But an ankle injury doesn't inhibit you from resistance training with your upper body or strengthening your core muscles. Give your injury plenty of time to mend, but keep the rest of your body on track while it's healing.
- **Ice.** Ice the affected area for 10–20 minutes at a time several times a day to reduce pain, swelling, and inflammation. It's best to cover the area being iced with a thin cloth or towel to prevent frostbite of the tissues.
- **Compression.** To help reduce swelling, wrap and compress the area with an Ace or other elastic bandage. Wrap it snugly enough to support the joint but not so tightly that it hinders circulation. If you feel numbness or tingling, you've done yourself up too tight.
- **Elevation.** Raise the injured area above your heart to help reduce swelling and pain. For example, lie on the couch with your twisted ankle propped up on a couple of pillows.

What do you use on an injury—ice or heat?
Always use ice after an acute injury such as an ankle sprain or on overuse injuries such as shin splints. This will help reduce pain and swelling and will allow the area to begin to heal. Never use heat on these injuries because it can increase the swelling and make things worse! Heat can be used on tight or irritated muscles that are in spasm, such as the lower back or neck, and can be an especially beneficial therapy before participating in activities that irritate those muscles. The heat gets blood moving into the area, oxygenating the tissues, loosening them up, and preparing them to work.

TYPICAL INJURIES

Here are some common sports injuries. Learn about them so you can prevent them!

Tendonitis
- **What is it?** The inflammation, over-stretching or tearing of a tendon (the tissue that connects muscle to bone).
- **Commonly occurs in:** Shoulders, knees, wrists, Achilles tendon, hips, elbows.
- **Cause:** Tendonitis is an overuse injury of soft tissue caused by repeated microtears, which cause pain and weaken the area. For example, if you're a right-handed tennis player, you might experience tendonitis in your right shoulder from repetitive hitting. Tendonitis can also occur as a result of aging; tendons lose elasticity as we get older and are more susceptible to injury.
- **Symptoms:** Pain, stiffness, swelling, or burning that surrounds the joint and tendon. Usually pain is worse following activity.
- **How long does it last?** Depending on the severity, tendonitis can last a few days or a few months.

- **Treatment:** Anti-inflammatories (ibuprofen or naproxen) and RICE. Physical therapy can also be helpful. In severe cases, cortisone may be injected directly into the tendon.
- **Prevention:** Regular stretching, cross-training, and proper warm-up and cool-down can help prevent tendonitis. Proper workout technique, a gradual increase in workout intensity, and good exercise form are also important for prevention.

Bursitis

- **What is it?** The inflammation of a bursa, a fluid-filled sac that cushions the area where muscles and tendons glide over bones. When inflamed, bursas lose their ability to "glide," causing pain.
- **Cause:** Bursitis is an overuse injury that usually comes from repetitive movements, either from a job (such as construction) or from a sport (throwing a baseball).
- **Commonly occurs in:** Knees, shoulders, elbows, hips.
- **Symptoms:** A burning sensation in the joint or surrounding area. Usually the pain is worse during and immediately after activity, or if pressure is applied to the area. The bursa might also swell, causing stiffness.
- **How long does it last?** With proper rest, bursitis can heal in a few days, provided you do not aggravate it again with more repetitive motions. If left untreated and constantly aggravated, bursitis can become chronic.
- **Treatment:** RICE, anti-inflammatories, and limited motion of the injured joint.
- **Prevention:** Learn proper exercise form and cross-train frequently to allow the injured part time to heal. Losing weight can often relieve bursitis in obese individuals.

Shin Splints

- **What is it?** Pain in the lower leg (tibia).
- **Causes:** Shin splits are an overuse injury that can be caused by a sudden increase in intensity, duration, or frequency of exercise, excessive tightness of the calves, exercising in old shoes, or participating in sports that involve sudden stops and starts, such as basketball and tennis.
- **Commonly occur in:** The lower leg.
- **Symptoms:** Tenderness, soreness, or pain along the inner part of your lower leg, even when not exercising; sometimes accompanied by mild swelling.
- **How long do they last?** Shin splits can last one to three weeks, depending on how severe they are.
- **Treatment:** RICE and anti-inflammatories.
- **Prevention:** Proper warm-up and cool-down, cross training, new shoes, flexibility training of the lower leg. If the problem persists, visit your podiatrist for some prescription orthotics.

Sprain

- **What is it?** A stretching or tearing of ligaments (the tissue that connects bones to bones).
- **Cause:** Sprains are acute injuries that occur when a joint is stretched in an unnatural way beyond its range of motion by an unusual force (such as twisting your ankle), or when physically hit in a contact sport such as football.
- **Commonly occurs in:** Ankles, wrists, knees.
- **Symptoms:** The affected area is usually tender to the touch, with pain, swelling, and bruising. The joint may be temporarily immobile or may feel unstable.
- **How long will it last?** Depending on the severity, a sprain can last anywhere from a few days to twelve weeks.

Athletic shoes have a life span of only six months or 500 miles! After that, the cushioning is inferior and you run a greater risk of joint pain and injury. If you've had your shoes for longer than six months or you've logged more than 500 miles in them (good job!), treat yourself to a new pair.

- **Treatment:** If you think you have a sprain, consult a physician. In the meantime, use RICE and anti-inflammatories.
- **Prevention:** Wear shoes and safety gear appropriate to your sport, warm up and cool down properly, and stretch frequently.

Strain (aka Pulled Muscle)
- **What is it?** An overstretching or tearing of muscle fibers.
- **Causes:** Strains can be acute or chronic (from overuse). Acute strains come from a stretching or tearing of a muscle caused by a trauma, such as lifting a heavy box improperly. Chronic strains can come from improper workout form, excessive physical activity, lack of flexibility, or repetitive overuse.
- **Commonly occurs in:** Hamstrings, lower back, quadriceps, neck.
- **Symptoms:** The affected part is usually stiff, sore, and difficult to move. This pain is often accompanied by swelling, cramping, discoloration, and muscle spasms.
- **How long will it last?** Usually between two and ten weeks. In the case of a severe tear, surgery may be required.
- **Treatment:** RICE, reduction of activity, and anti-inflammatories. Physical therapy can also help.
- **Prevention:** Proper warm-up and cool-down, regular flexibility training, proper workout form, and gradual workout progression.

Blister
- **What is it?** A painful, fluid-filled area that occurs when the surface layer of skin, irritated by friction, becomes separated from the lower layer. The space between layers fills with fluid called serum.
- **Causes:** Blisters are commonly the result of poorly fitting athletic shoes or clothing that causes friction with the skin.
- **Commonly occur on:** Hands and feet.
- **Symptoms:** A raised, fluid-filled area of skin that is painful to the touch and is easily irritated by shoes or clothing.
- **How long will it last?** Small blisters usually heal on their own in a few days; larger ones may take up to a week.
- **Treatment:** It's best to leave blisters alone. The fluid inside gets reabsorbed, so simply cover them with a bandage until they heal. If a blister breaks, wash it with soap and water, then apply a bandage.
- **Prevention:** Minimize friction by wearing proper footwear and soft, absorbent socks made from synthetic fibers.

Stress Fracture
- **What is it?** Tiny cracks in bones.
- **Causes:** Stress fractures can be caused by repeated pounding, such as running on pavement, or because of a sudden increase in exercise intensity or duration, putting a lot of stress on muscles and joints.
- **Commonly occur in:** Bones of the lower leg and feet.
- **Symptoms:** Pain that increases with activity, pain while at rest, swelling, and areas that are painful to the touch.
- **How long will it last?** Anywhere from four weeks to four months, depending on the severity of the fracture.
- **Treatment:** Long periods of rest are usually needed, along with a modification of activity. Regular RICE treatment is also beneficial.
- **Prevention:** Increase your workout intensity, duration, and frequency gradually; wear proper shoes; and cross-train often.

PAIN BEFORE GAIN

You might notice that one or two days after you work out, you're sore. This post-workout pain is called delayed-onset muscle soreness, or DOMS for short. DOMS is thought to occur because of microscopic tears in the muscle tissue as a result of exercise. You may initially mistake DOMS for an injury, but don't worry—DOMS is normal and does not indicate a problem; this soreness means only that you've worked out hard and your body is repairing and rebuilding itself to be stronger and better than it was before. Typically DOMS lasts one to three days and gradually dissipates. Gently stretching the sore areas a few times a day can help accelerate healing and alleviate stiffness and soreness. Light cardio work can also alleviate some soreness, as it gets blood flowing into the affected areas, helping remove wastes and oxygenate regenerating cells. Regular flexibility training and proper warm-up and cool-down can help prevent DOMS, but the best cure for DOMS is time. Wait a few days, and it will go away. If it doesn't go away, you've got something else going on.

BURNING QUESTION

How do I tell if I have DOMS or a more serious injury? DOMS occurs a few hours after you're done working out and typically lasts one to three days. Usually the soreness is worst on the second day—at least it is for me! But it usually lightens up after that and should be completely gone within a week. If you have a nagging ache or pain that lasts longer than a week, keep your eye on it to make sure it's not an overuse injury. Acute injuries such as tears, sprains, and strains are painful right away—believe me, you'll know when you've got one! I tore my

Achilles tendon in 2001, and let me tell you, I knew right away something bad had happened! There was a loud popping noise, followed by a lot of swelling. Within fifteen minutes, I couldn't move my foot. In fact, I had to drive my stick-shift car to the doctor's office using my emergency brake because I could not use the clutch. (Looking back, I wonder why I didn't call a cab; stubbornness, I suppose!) In any case, if one of these injuries occurs to you, stop exercising at once, apply RICE, and get to a doctor right away. (And for heaven's sake, call a cab!) On a positive note, I didn't let this injury sideline me. I started to write, and I discovered the benefits of Pilates, yoga, and other flexibility training.

INJURY PREVENTION

While these injuries sound daunting, there are several ways you can prevent them. All it takes is a little foresight and some dedication to keep yourself healthy and injury free!

- **Always warm up.** As I said before, your muscles are like taffy—when they are warmer, they are more flexible and less likely to snap, stretch, or tear.
- **Always cool down and stretch.** Slowly allow your body to return to a normal resting state after a workout, and follow up with a flexibility routine to improve your range of motion.
- **Wear proper safety equipment for sports.** Helmets, shin guards, mouth guards, protective padding, and other safety gear can help prevent acute injuries.
- **Wear proper clothing and shoes.** To prevent chafing and blisters, wear clothing appropriate for your activity. If your shoes are old and worn out, replace them to decrease wear and tear on your joints and muscles.

Medi-alerts

- Call your doctor if swelling does not go down within two days, the area becomes red, you develop a fever, or the pain lasts more than a week. This indicates a more serious condition!

- Seek medical attention if you hear a "popping" sound at the time of injury; you can't put your weight on the injured joint; or the pain, swelling, and stiffness do not improve within three days.

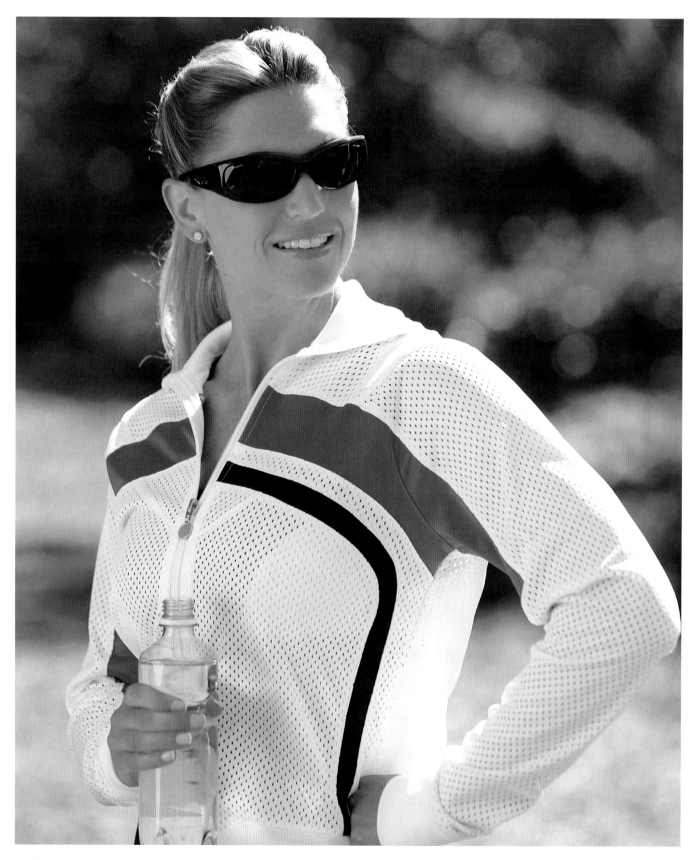

- **Gradually increase your workout time, frequency, and intensity.** Think of workout progression as bricklaying: You have to carefully lay the foundation and stack the bricks slowly to make the walls before you put on the roof. The same goes for your workouts. You have to lay a solid foundation of strength, endurance, and flexibility before you go out and run a 10K. If you try to do too much too soon, you're setting yourself up for injury.
- **Use proper workout form.** Proper form will keep your joints lined up correctly, decreasing your chance for injury.
- **Cross-train with a variety of activities.** Use your muscles in different ways with a variety of exercises, sports, and cardio activities to prevent overuse injuries and keep you from getting bored!
- **Take days off.** Remember that your Rest Days are as important as your training days. Give your body enough time to rest and repair to better prevent overuse injuries.
- **Get enough sleep.** While you're sleeping, your body produces hormones that repair and rebuild tissues, helping you lose weight, change your shape, and improve your body composition. Get at least seven to nine hours of quality, uninterrupted sleep every night, especially when starting a new fitness program.

SUMMARY

Even the best athletes get injured from time to time, but with diligent planning and proper prevention measures, you can greatly reduce your chances for injury. If you do get injured, apply RICE, contact your physician, and follow his or her instructions to heal quickly and get back to your program as soon as possible.

TOO WOUND UP TO SLEEP?

TRY THESE TIPS

- **Read a book.** Reading is a good way to distract your mind from your day's events.
- **Drink a hot beverage.** Warmth is soothing and will promote drowsiness and relaxation. Certain kinds of tea such as chamomile and kava kava also contain relaxing herbs.
- **Change your workout time.** Sometimes an evening workout can wake you up too much. See whether working out in the morning instead makes a difference in your sleeping pattern.
- **Go decaf after noon.** The less caffeine you ingest in the afternoons and evenings, the better your sleep pattern will be.

HOMEWORK

1. Check your shoes for excessive wear. If they look worn and torn, buy yourself a new pair to prevent overuse injuries such as stress fractures, shin splints, and bursitis.
2. Check your socks for excessive wear. If they look threadbare, buy some new ones to prevent blisters.
3. Today and for the rest of this week, bring your lunch to work, and bring snacks with you when you're out and about for long periods of time. To read more about the importance of being prepared with your own snacks and meals, turn to page 218!

Extra Credit

Always be prepared. Buy yourself a few Ace bandages, some cold packs, a few anti-inflammatories, and a small first aid kit to keep handy in case of injury.

Fun Fact
When you exercise, you sleep better!

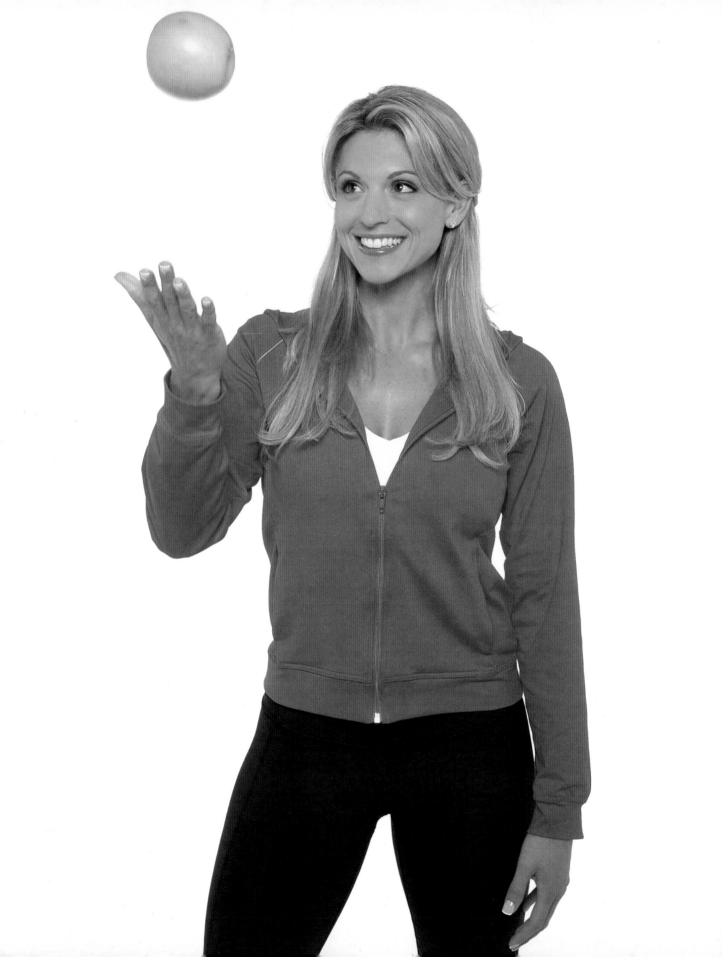

Your Nutrition

MUCH OF YOUR WEIGHT-LOSS BATTLE will go down in the kitchen! Here's a nifty analogy for you: If you feed a racehorse only sugar cubes, he'll never win a race because he doesn't have adequate fuel. But if you feed him quality oats, hay, and plenty of fresh water, he'll be strong and healthy and will win any race he enters. The same goes for your body. If you feed it fast food, processed snacks, and empty sugar calories, even if you're exercising, you'll see very few gains. But if you feed your body high-quality complex carbs, lean proteins, and healthy fats, you'll be able to meet any goals you set.

The *Your Body, Your Life* nutritional plan is not a quick-fix gimmick but rather a way of eating designed for longevity, a plan you can use for the rest of your life. What you learn in this section will give you all the tools you need to succeed with all your fitness and weight-loss goals.

CHAPTER 11

The Bad Fad

*T*his is the latest, greatest, weight-loss *diet, guaranteed to melt away fat and cellulite and give you the body you've always wanted in less time than it takes to tie your shoes!!*

You can't pick up a magazine or watch television these days without being bombarded by quick-fix diet ads like these. Such advertorial pitches are remarkably convincing to the average Joe, since they're usually backed by the testimony of a doctor or a "success story," someone who tried the diet and easily lost enormous amounts of weight. But if you look carefully at the small print, there is always a disclaimer, such as "Results not typical" or "Used in conjunction with healthy eating and exercise." Because truthfully, no one can lose weight and get healthy using only a fad diet; there has to be a balance of healthful nutrition and exercise in order to lose weight and keep it off. When you're done with this chapter, you'll be an expert on fad diets, what they

do and don't do for your body, and how they can affect your physical and emotional health.

WHAT IS A FAD DIET?

Fad diets are nothing more than bogus schemes designed to cause dramatic and rapid weight loss for desperate dieters. They are monotonous, unrealistic, and restrictive and only teach you how to set outrageous boundaries on your eating. None of them teach you how to balance your nutrition to keep the weight off once you've lost it; what's more, fads don't offer any guidelines for exercise, a dead giveaway that they are bogus. Weight loss is a game of calories in versus calories out, and the only way to expend calories and burn off true body fat is with a balanced nutrition formula and a regular exercise plan.

Even though this explanation prob-ably makes complete sense to most of you, I can hear your thoughts right now—*I have to get in shape for a wedding next month, and fast, temporary weight loss sounds great!* This is the exact thought process that perpetuates this multibillion-dollar industry and keeps fad diets alive and thriving. But in reality, the quick fix you'll get now from crash dieting will do you way more harm than good.

FAD DIETS: BREAKDOWN

Most fads force the body to lose weight in one of three ways: through elimination of one or more food groups, through severe calorie restriction, or through the use of stimulant pills or drinks.

Elimination Diets

Many fads eliminate one or more types of foods, such as fruit, meat, carbohydrates, or fats. To me, these are the worst types of fads. They drill it into your brain that certain foods are "forbidden," at the same time offering no information about how to balance your nutrition properly. Over the long term, elimination diets can cause vitamin and mineral deficiency, nausea, dizziness, weakness, constipation, hair loss, and irritability. Moreover, they set you up for absolute failure once you're done with the diet; your craving and desire for those "forbidden" foods usually causes you to binge on them when you go back to normal eating, causing weight gain and emotional distress.

> ## HOW TO IDENTIFY A FAD DIET
> - It sounds too good to be true.
> - It makes outlandish promises.
> - It "guarantees" extreme weight loss in a short period of time.
> - It excludes one or more foods.
> - It overemphasizes one or more foods.
> - It categorizes foods into "good" and "bad" lists.
> - It severely restricts calories to fewer than 1,200 a day.
> - It claims you can "trick" your body in some way.
> - It does not contain a program of regular exercise.

The Low-Carb Craze

The most popular type of elimination diet these days is the low-carbohydrate diet. Many of my clients have tried this type of diet, not only because of dramatic "weight" loss during the first week, but also because they were able to eat their vice foods, such as butter, sour cream, egg yolks, and fatty meats, without feeling guilty. Still, low-carb dieters often lose up to 10 pounds in the first week without really trying. But what did they lose? Was it fat? No. Mostly it was water.

During the first week of a carb-restrictive diet, your body converts the carbohydrates and glycogen (stored energy) left in your system into glucose (blood sugar), the energy used to run your

Fad Facts

- Since many low-carb dieters don't restrict their intake of proteins and fats, their total caloric intake typically exceeds their daily needs, further decreasing their chances for real weight loss.

- For every pound of lean tissue you lose through crash dieting, you burn 30–50 fewer calories per day!

metabolism, brain, and other vital systems. Since glycogen is stored in the muscles and liver with three to four times its weight in water, when you break down and use a pound of glycogen, you'll also eliminate 3 to 4 pounds of water through the urine. Many people perceive this as weight loss, but it's simply metabolic dehydration. Once the glycogen is gone, you'll feel sluggish, tired, distracted, and irritable as your body tries to use fat as its primary fuel source, putting a huge strain on your kidneys. Your brain demands glucose to function, but since glucose comes from carbohydrates—which you're not eating—your brain gets crabby. In addition to feeling rotten and overloading your kidneys, "weight" loss slows dramatically and sometimes even stops after the first two weeks. There is no more excess water to excrete, and your body is now being forced to use body fat as fuel, which would be great if you could actually keep it up! But realistically, no one can. Human beings need carbohydrates to function properly—period.

Here is the ugly underbelly of this sort of diet that no one ever tells you about: Once you go off the diet and return to eating carbs, your body experiences a huge rebound. Your cells, starved for glucose, gorge themselves, and hence take on water to help digest the glucose for energy. Severe bloating often occurs, which many depressed dieters perceive as weight gain. This causes feelings of failure and a cavalier attitude toward eating; dieters think, *This diet didn't work either, so who cares if I eat a whole pizza? I'm doomed anyhow.* In addition, the sudden influx of glucose can cause headaches, stomachaches, and intestinal distress.

All in all, low-carb diets and elimination diets are for the birds! Human beings

were designed to eat a variety of foods from all five food groups. Elimination of one or more of these groups goes against the balance of nature.

BURNING QUESTION

What's the deal with protein drinks and meal replacement shakes? Protein drinks and meal-replacement shakes are not the same thing. Protein drinks are usually low-calorie, high-protein powders that, when blended with water or skim milk, make great post-workout meals or snacks for people on the go. Meal-replacement shakes, on the other hand, are usually high-calorie, premixed drinks that contain moderate protein, a lot of carbs, and some fat. They are designed to "replace" a meal if you're too busy to stop and eat or if you're dieting and avoiding certain foods. Both kinds of products may contain added ingredients that are not good for weight loss, so always read the label. Avoid products that contain excessive amounts of sugar, fat, and other hidden calories. Remember, losing weight is a game of calories in versus calories out; it's easy to drink your meal, but it's just as easy to overdrink your meal! Also remember that no shake is a substitute for real food. They are supplements, meaning they should support a healthy eating plan and not comprise its entirety.

Caloric Restriction (aka "Crash" Dieting)

Many fads rely on severe caloric restriction to force the body to lose weight, some promoting a daily intake of fewer than 1,000 calories a day! That's just plain starvation, and if that's your bag, sign up for *Survivor*! At least you'll have a shot at a million dollars in the end.

The nickname for these diets—"crash diets"—is amazingly appropriate because that is exactly what happens to your metabolism—it crashes and burns! If your body is not receiving adequate fuel, it goes into a starvation mode, hoarding any calories taken in and storing them as body fat. Your body becomes resistant and unwilling to release those stored calories for use as fuel for fear of going through another long stretch of starvation, so in order to create glucose to fuel the body and brain, the body turns to protein. Protein is much easier to break down than fat, and as you already know, your body is holding on to that fat for dear life, since it has no idea how long you're going to be "starving." So guess where it gets the protein to make the glucose? Your muscles! You'll literally cannibalize your muscle tissues for use as fuel instead of fat if you're not taking in enough calories. If you continue a pattern of calorie-restrictive diets or stay on one of these plans for an extended period of time, your body eventually resets its basal metabolic rate to a lower level than it was at before. It adapts, becomes more efficient, and functions day to day on fewer calories than it needed previously, making it even more difficult for you to lose weight!

Calorie-restrictive diets can also perpetuate a habit of bingeing. Once dieters are done with the program, they eat anything and everything they were denied while on the diet, and then some. Your body wants the calories physically as much as you want them mentally, but since your body takes a bit longer to understand that you're done "starving," it continues to hoard calories, storing them as more body fat. Therefore, a repeated pattern of calorie-restrictive diets will in fact make you fatter rather than skinnier!

To lose weight, you do have to limit your caloric intake, but in a healthy way. You have to eat enough calories to fuel your metabolism during the day and enable you to function, but you should be eating few enough to encourage your body to use fat weight as fuel.

Pills and Teas

Never in the history of mankind has someone lost weight solely because of a pill, drink, or tea. I do believe some products are useful as energy boosters and workout enhancers, and may help you lose weight when combined with good nutrition and a solid exercise plan. But none of them will magically take you from a size 12 to a size 2, no matter how convincing the ads.

Many "dieter's teas" and weight-loss pills contain stimulant laxatives, which work in the gastrointestinal tract to expel waste. Often, this expulsion occurs quickly, before your body has a chance to extract all the nutrients it needs from the food. Overuse or continual use of laxatives can cause resistance to the product, damage to the intestines, kidney stones, and in extreme cases kidney failure. Some laxatives can also cause dehydration, as they encourage the intestines to take in water. My point is that these teas are not helping you lose fat weight; they're only emptying your bowels so it seems like you're losing weight.

The other main ingredient in many over-the-counter pills and teas is a stimulant, such as highly concentrated amounts of synthetic caffeine or herbal stimulants such as guarana, green tea, or kola nut. These stimulants are supposed to increase your metabolism while decreasing your desire for food. Some people like the boost of energy they get

CLIENT CORNER

FAD FREAK-OUT, BY JENNIFER

I have been obese since I was seven years old. My first experience with an organized diet plan was in junior high school when my mother took me to Weight Watchers with her. I was excited about the promised weight loss, but since the payoff wasn't immediate, I quickly lost interest. Truthfully, I didn't get much out of the program, except the proclivity to obsess even more about my weight. This led me to try all sorts of fad diets—including some plan that had me eating nothing but carrots and turned my skin orange! It sounds silly, but I had no idea these diets were fads. I really thought they were the answer I was looking for. There were always these incredible testimonials to back them up, and I thought, *It worked for those people, why not me?*

But the thing is, nothing worked. I could not keep up with the regimented guidelines of the fads, and the second I declared my diet was done, I binged on everything I had been denied during that time. I gained back all the weight I had lost and then some. With each diet I became more bitter and my sense of humor more sarcastic. I was highly critical of myself, and my negative self-talk was out of control. But still, I tried more diets. It was easier to invest short term in a fad than it was to invest long term in myself.

What none of these programs gave me was what I finally found with Kim—balance. There has to be a balance of nutritional elements in your diet—no outlandish restrictions, no points, no pills—just balanced, wholesome meals made with fresh ingredients and whole foods. What's more, fads don't educate you about the importance of exercise. It's a combination of healthy habits—solid nutrition and consistent exercise—that you've got to adopt for a lifetime in order to lose weight and keep it off forever.

from pills such as these, while others feel like they are having a heart attack. Depending on your sensitivity to these types of ingredients, you may experience jitteriness, loss of concentration, irritability, and even heart palpitations in extreme cases. Prescription appetite suppressants and weight-loss drugs also contain stimulants and other chemicals that "speed" you up, decrease your desire for food, or even make food taste bad. But unless you're going to take these pills for life, you're probably going to experience weight gain when you go off them; you've still learned nothing about balanced nutrition and will likely go right back to your old pre-pill habits.

My advice remains the same: No pill replaces good old-fashioned nutritional know-how, and nothing is better for losing weight and keeping it off than balanced diet and exercise.

BURNING QUESTION

Should I take a vitamin pill? The debate over whether or not human beings need to supplement with vitamin pills is a hot-button issue. Those opposed claim we should be able to get all the vitamins necessary from food; those in favor argue that the soil has become depleted and our produce is of lower quality than it was a decade ago. To make up for the paucity of vitamins in the foods we eat, they argue that we should take a vitamin pill to ensure we're getting everything we need. Personally, I am all for taking a good multivitamin and mineral supplement once a day. At most, you're getting all the nutrients you need to live and function; at the least, you have expensive urine. And since a standard, store-brand multivitamin costs only about fifty bucks a year, that's pretty cheap health insurance, if you ask me!

GETTING MENTAL OVER FADS

I can safely say that all of my clients have tried one or more fad diets in their lifetime, and these are not stupid people! They are accountants, lawyers, fighter pilots, engineers—how could such smart people get sucked in by such stupid claims? Because they wanted to. Across the board, my clients tell me the fad sounded easy and achievable. They were encouraged because they would not have to work hard and would be guaranteed dramatic results in a short period of time.

In a way, I can understand this willing dupe. Losing weight is a difficult challenge to face, especially if you've got 40, 50, 100, or more pounds to lose. The task seems daunting, even impossible, and it's easy to see where you would want to accomplish it in the fastest way possible. But honestly, it didn't take you two weeks to gain 30 pounds—what makes you think you can lose 30 pounds in two weeks? I don't believe people think these diets are a lasting way of life. Rather, they feel desperate and impatient and are willing to try anything that promises weight loss quickly. But whether they choose to try a fad because of desperation, laziness, or gullibility does not matter; what does matter is that no fad worked for them. Invariably, once they returned to normal eating patterns, they gained back every pound they lost, and then some. What's worse, they didn't learn one darn thing about nutrition and ended up more confused than ever about healthy eating.

SUMMARY

Fad diets do you more harm than good over the long term. They stress your body physically, causing your weight to yo-yo and wreaking havoc on your metabolism and body composition. They also stress you mentally, fostering a burgeoning sense of failure and self-loathing as you fail time and again at these diets. Nothing beats solid, sensible nutrition and regular exer-cise when it comes to losing weight and keeping it off, no matter what the ads say!

HOMEWORK

1. Read as many diet pill and supplement ads as you can and look closely at the fine print. What do you see?
2. Think back to any fad diet you might have tried yourself. Reread this chapter and then deduce why that fad did not work for you.
3. Today and for the rest of this week, cook yourself or your family a healthy dinner. For recipe suggestions, turn to Chapter 16!

Fad Fact
Just because a product is labeled "all natural" does not mean it's good for you! Case in point: DDT, cigarettes, and cocaine all contain natural ingredients . . . 'nuf said!

CHAPTER 12

Back to Basics

Fun Facts

- After water, protein makes up the largest portion of your body weight. This includes muscles, ligaments, tendons, organs, glands, nails, and hair!

- It takes almost twice the energy to digest protein as it does to digest carbohydrates!

Last week, I watched a bunch of daytime talk shows to see what kind of nutritional information was being aired these days, and I have to tell you, I was amazed. Every program had a different doctor or nutritional "guru" pushing some crazy diet or other that they swore was the key to lasting weight loss. From the raw-food diet to the caveman diet, each "expert" pitched a different spiel about proper nutrition, each often contradicting the other in the process. Even the nightly news that week featured breaking stories about nutritional studies proving (or disproving) that certain foods were good (or bad) for you. Many of these stories refuted current nutritional beliefs. With all this conflicting information, where is the truth? Who is right? What to believe? Nutrition has become unnecessarily complicated, and I can totally understand why people are getting frustrated, throwing their hands in the air and saying, *Forget it!*

But there is no reason nutrition should be so frustrating; in this chapter we'll get back to basics—good old-fashioned food basics like the ones you learned in grade school. Yes, it's that simple. Knowing these basics will enable you to formulate a diet to work with your lifestyle, offering you an opportunity for lasting weight loss. No fancy gimmicks or outrageous diet plans here—just good, solid, *truthful* information about the foods you eat and what they do and don't do for your body.

The most basic nutritional elements are proteins, carbohydrates, and fats. Each of your meals should contain all three of these elements for you to lose weight and thrive. Let's start there!

PROTEIN

Protein is broken down by the body into amino acids, which are used to build muscle, grow hair, manufacture hormones, form hemoglobin, create enzymes, and maintain the health of internal organs. Protein also slows the movement of food from the stomach to the intestine, making you feel satisfied for a longer period of

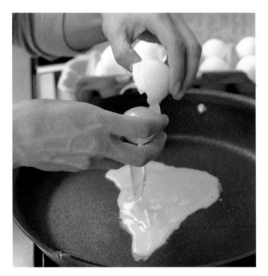

Egg whites are a great, inexpensive source of complete protein!

time after eating. Because the body does not store amino acids, you must eat them on a daily basis, and each of your meals should contain a protein.

Proteins are subdivided into one of two groups depending on how many amino acids they contain. *Complete* proteins contain the full spectrum of amino acids the body needs to function properly. These include animal proteins such as meat, poultry, fish, eggs, dairy, and cheese. *Incomplete* proteins contain only some of the essential amino acids and should be eaten in combination with other incomplete proteins to get all the

PROTEIN IN A NUTSHELL

PROTEIN BASICS

- Promotes a feeling of fullness (satiety)
- Builds muscles, tissues, ligaments, bones, hair, and nails
- Helps manufacture hormones, hemoglobin, and enzymes
- Provides energy
- Stabilizes blood sugar
- Contains 4 calories per gram
- Can be either complete or incomplete

TEN GREAT PROTEINS

- lean beef
- lean pork chops
- 99 percent fat-free ground turkey or beef
- low- or no-fat cottage cheese or string cheese
- skinless chicken breasts
- sushi or sashimi
- shellfish (shrimp, lobster, mussels, clams)
- egg whites
- low-fat tofu
- low-fat protein shakes

TEN UNDESIRABLE PROTEINS

- high-fat ground beef (fat content ›93 percent)
- full-fat milk
- full-fat hard cheese and cream cheeses
- bacon
- high-fat tofu
- chicken wings or other dark poultry meats
- roasted duck
- spare ribs
- full-fat refried beans
- oil-roasted nuts

TEN GREAT VEGETARIAN PROTEINS

- beans/legumes
- low-fat tofu
- low-fat cottage cheese
- low-fat hard cheese
- skim milk or fat-free soy milk
- raw or dry-roasted nuts and seeds
- all-natural raw nut butters
- hummus
- quinoa
- tempeh

Rule of Thumb

- Remove the skin from any meat, fish, or poultry product to decrease the fat content of a meal!

- Avoid purchasing ground meat where the fat content is not clearly indicated! These products often contain meat by-products (gristle, tendons, ligaments) and tons of fat.

- Most vegetarian proteins are incomplete. Combine them in a meal to derive the most nutrition!

amino acids needed for optimal health. These include soy products, legumes, and whole grains.

Because complete proteins usually come from animal sources, be aware of their fat content. Always choose the lowest-fat options of ground meats, cheeses, and other dairy items, and trim away excess fat and skin from roasts, poultry, and beef products.

CARBOHYDRATES

Contrary to popular belief, carbohydrates are not evil! They are a necessary and important nutrient for the human body. Carbs are the number one source of energy used by the body to fuel the metabolism, nervous system, and brain function. To lose fat, you've got to eat carbohydrates!

Carbohydrates are broken down by the body into glucose (blood sugar), which is either used by cells for fuel or stored in the liver and muscles as glycogen. But here is the tricky part: Excess glucose can also be stored in the body as fat. How do you avoid this problem? Choose your carbs wisely.

Carbohydrates fall into two categories: simple and complex. Simple carbs are broken down quickly into glucose, causing a sharp spike in blood sugar and a subsequent increase in insulin production. Insulin "mops up" glucose from the blood, taking it to cells for use as fuel, storing it as glycogen, or, if there is an excess, storing it as body fat. (Sometimes this extra insulin even swabs up too much glucose, resulting in hunger pangs soon after eating!) Complex carbohydrates take longer to break down and do not cause a sharp spike in blood sugar. They contain more fiber than simple carbs, keeping you fuller longer and providing a more even release of glucose and insulin into the

bloodstream. When you eat more complex carbs, you're less likely to store those calories as body fat because your body is better able to handle the steady influx of blood sugar.

The Glycemic Index

The glycemic index (GI) shows the rate at which carbohydrates break down into glucose in the body. Straight glucose has been given the highest number on the scale (100), and other foods are rated in comparison. High-glycemic (simple) carbs fall closer to 100 than low-glycemic (complex) carbs and are usually refined, manufactured products that contain added sugar and little fiber, such as pasta, white bread, soda, and fruit juice. These are considered fast-acting carbohydrates because they break down quickly, causing a rapid rise in blood sugar. Low-glycemic carbs rate lower on the scale and are typically whole foods that contain a lot of fiber and some protein, such as brown rice, vegetables, beans, and oatmeal. The closer to the number 1 the item falls, the slower acting it is, releasing glucose into the bloodstream at a steady rate, providing the brain and body with a prolonged and constant energy level.

When to Eat Which Carbs

To maintain a healthy body and mind, you've got to eat a wide variety of carbs, both high and low glycemic. To properly fuel your metabolism and your workouts while discouraging the storage of body fat, you've got to time your carbs carefully. I recommend eating moderate- and higher-glycemic (starchy) carbs earlier in the day, and lower-glycemic (fibrous) carbs in the afternoon and evening. The starchy carbs provide you with sustained energy, help maintain stable blood sugar levels, and fuel your workouts. Having fibrous carbs

The Glycemic Index
Ratings of a few common foods

Food	Rating
Peanuts	13
Yogurt, plain	14
Soy beans	15
Cherries	22
Black beans	30
Skim milk	32
Apples	38
Oranges	43
Carrots	49
Chocolate	49
Brown rice	50
Sweet potatoes	52
Bananas	56
Honey	62
Table sugar	64
Raisins	64
Cola	65
Wheat bread	68
Corn chips	72
Pretzels	83
Red potatoes	93
Glucose	100

CARBOHYDRATES IN A NUTSHELL

CARBOHYDRATES BASICS
- All carbs are broken down into glucose
- Carbs provide energy to the body and brain
- Simple carbs are quickly broken down into glucose
- Complex carbs take longer to break down
- Complex carbs provide fiber as well as energy
- The glycemic index indicates how quickly a food is broken down into glucose
- Carbohydrates contain 4 calories per gram
- Eat higher-glycemic carbs earlier in the day and lower-glycemic carbs in the afternoon and evening

TEN SIMPLE (HIGHER-GLYCEMIC) CARBS
- table sugar
- soft drinks
- fruit juice
- white bread
- crackers
- rice cakes
- honey, jelly, jam, syrup
- mashed potatoes
- white rice
- corn flakes

TEN COMPLEX (LOWER-GLYCEMIC) CARBS
- yams
- brown or wild rice
- sweet potatoes
- whole-grain bread
- green, leafy vegetables (broccoli, spinach, kale, arugula)
- whole raw or dried fruits
- oatmeal
- oat or wheat bran
- beans
- root vegetables (carrots, parsnips, turnips)

such as vegetables at night helps move things along in the gut and will cut back on the likelihood that you'll store excess glucose as fat.

And guess what—you can still eat bread, pasta, and potatoes! Just time these things correctly. The best time to eat simple carbs like these is after a workout when you have depleted your blood sugar and stored glycogen. Your body wants to replenish these right away, so calories eaten

Fun Fact
The brain is picky: It will use only glucose as fuel! Not protein, not fat; only glucose.

- Dextrose, maltodextrose, fructose, high-fructose corn syrup, corn syrup, malt syrup, and sucrose are all aliases for sugar! Any product containing these ingredients will rate higher on the glycemic index.

- The more naturally colorful and textured your carbohydrate, the better it is for you!

Fun Fact

Research suggests that eating 6 ounces per week of fatty fish (salmon, herring, mackerel, anchovies, or sardines) may reduce the risk of fatal heart disease by 36 percent!

within an hour of working out will go mostly toward replacing depleted muscle and liver glycogen stores and repairing muscle tissue instead of being stored as fat. You can also eat higher-glycemic foods in combination with a protein or fat to slow their effect on blood sugar. For instance, a baked potato eaten with a piece of chicken will cause a less dramatic blood sugar spike than a baked potato eaten alone.

FAT

Dietary fat is not the same as body fat, and though you might swear you see that piece of fudge pop up on your hindquarters an hour after eating it, things don't really work that way! Fat has the highest caloric concentration per gram (9 calories per gram) and provides tons of energy when it's used as fuel, but because it's so calorie dense it is also very easy to overeat. Since excess calories (of any kind!) are usually stored as body fat, you've got to control your fat intake to prevent that from happening. All that being said, however, you still need to eat fat. Fat is broken down by the body into fatty acids, which support the reproductive, nervous, and immune systems and give you healthy bones, joints, skin, and hair. Fats also help the body absorb vitamins A, D, E, and K and build cell membranes.

Like carbs, not all fats are created equal. Saturated fats occur naturally in animal products such as meat, whole-milk dairy products, poultry skin, and egg yolks, and in some plant foods such as coconuts, palm oil, and coconut oil. Research has shown that these fats have a tendency to be "stored" rather than used as fuel, so limit your intake of these fats as much as possible. Saturated and trans fats have also been linked to an increased risk

for heart disease, high blood pressure, high cholesterol, obesity, and type 2 diabetes. They also raise the bad (LDL) cholesterol in the bloodstream while depleting the good (HDL) cholesterol. All the more reason to avoid them!

Unsaturated fats, however, have the opposite effect on the body. They reduce the risk of those same diseases, decrease LDL cholesterol, and increase HDL cholesterol. Unsaturated fats are usually a liquid at room temperature and are found in plant foods such as olive oil, flaxseeds, peanuts, and canola oil, as well as in fish such as salmon, halibut, albacore, and light chunk tuna. Fish and fish oils also contain omega-3 fatty acids, which have been associated with a lowered risk of coronary heart disease.

BURNING QUESTION

What are trans fats? Trans fats are basically vegetable fats that have been altered chemically in a process known as hydrogenation. This process takes a normally liquid substance and transforms it into a solid at room temperature, making it more stable for product shelf life but more dangerous for your body. Because trans fats are not natural, they are difficult for your body to digest. They cause all kinds of internal problems, including lowering your immune response, elevating your cholesterol, and increasing your blood lipoprotein levels. They are also linked to several nasty diseases, including coronary artery disease, stroke, diabetes, and heart attacks. Yes, these are the fats directly responsible for clogging your arteries! Think of a sink: Over time, gunk such as bacon grease, butter, and frying oil accumulates in the pipes and hardens up, blocking the pipes. This is the same way trans (and saturated) fats act in your body.

They collect along the lining of your arteries, clogging them up and constricting the blood flow to the body and the brain. Over time, this accumulation of fats can lead to heart attacks, ischemia, and stroke.

Trans fats are found in commercially prepared baked goods (donuts, cakes, cookies, pastries, pies), margarine, fried foods, crackers, icing, chips, even microwave popcorn. As of January 1, 2006, manufacturers are required to list trans fats on their labels. Look for it right underneath "saturated fats" on the nutritional chart on the packaging. If the product does not have such a chart, look for trans fat aliases in the ingredients such as partially hydrogenated vegetable oil, hydrogenated oil, or vegetable shortening. The higher up on the list of ingredients these appear, the more of them are contained in the product.

SUMMARY

See, that wasn't so bad, was it? I hope this cleared up some of the confusion regarding proper nutrition. As you've learned, it doesn't have to be complicated or horrifying. Just stick with the most natural, whole foods you can find and eat a balance from the three macronutrient food groups, and you'll be on your way toward better health and ultimate weight loss!

HOMEWORK

1. Grab a can of soup, a box of cookies, or a package of chips out of your kitchen cabinet and inspect the list of ingredients. How much protein, carbs, and fats are in there? Are there any ingredients you don't recognize? Are there any trans fats? Write down the ingredients you think are suspicious and look them up.
2. Get out the food log you kept for a whole week back in Chapter 5. Look through it carefully and note how much of each macronutrient you are taking in each day. Keep this journal out and in mind for when you read the section on portion control in Chapter 14.
3. Today and for the rest of the week get more activity in your daily routine. Park in the farthest space in the parking lot; take the stairs at work; walk to do short errands instead of driving. To read more about the importance of increasing your daily activity, turn to page 26!

DIETARY FAT IN A NUTSHELL

DIETARY FAT BASICS

- Helps the body absorb vitamins A, D, E, and K
- Is a component of cell membranes
- Contains 9 calories per gram
- Is not the same as body fat
- Saturated and trans fats are associated with high risk of disease
- Unsaturated fats are associated with disease prevention
- Supports the reproductive, nervous, and immune systems
- Contributes to the health of bones, skin, joints, and hair

TEN GREAT FATS

- avocado
- raw nuts (almonds, cashews, peanuts)
- all-natural nut butters
- flaxseeds or flaxseed oil
- olive oil
- fish oil
- olives
- peanut oil
- fatty fish (salmon, mackerel, herring)
- shellfish (crab, shrimp, lobster)

TEN NOT-SO-GREAT FATS

- butter and margarine (stick and spread)
- egg yolks
- lard
- Palm oil
- hydrogenated oils
- full-fat mayonnaise
- ice cream
- coconuts/coconut milk and oil
- vegetable shortening
- cream cheese

Rule of Thumb

- The more natural and unprocessed the source of your dietary fat, the better it is for you!

- With the exception of nuts and avocados, if a fat is solid at room temperature, such as butter or margarine, it's not good for you!

CHAPTER 13

Beyond the Basics

Now that you're an expert on macronutrients, we're going one step farther, because not everything fits into a neat little category! This is where many people get confused, because they get all caught up in the nitpicky details and forget the basics. But the basics do not change, even given the information in this chapter: You will still need to eat a balance of protein, carbs, and fat to maintain a healthy body and lose weight.

This chapter simply gives you additional info on fiber, water, alcohol, sweets, and sodium, as well as fat-free and sugar-free foods to help accelerate your weight-loss process. While the macronutrients may be the three main base players in the nutrition baseball field, items such as water, "free" foods, and fiber support the outfield, while alcohol, sweets, and sodium play for the other team. Understanding and practicing what you learn in this chapter will maximize your progress and help you hit a home run with all your goals!

FIBER
Dietary fiber is the indigestible complex carbohydrate found in fresh vegetables, fresh and dried fruits, beans, seeds, and whole-grain cereals and breads. There are two kinds of fiber: insoluble and soluble. Insoluble fiber adds bulk to your meals, helping promote a feeling of fullness and digestive regularity, which is associated with reduced risk for certain types of cancers. This type of fiber is found in edible fruit peels (apples, pears, plums), whole wheat, carrots, celery, and nuts. Soluble fiber combines with water to create a sort of "gel," which slows the release of sugar into the bloodstream and traps and eliminates excess cholesterol from the body. This type of fiber is found in oats, bananas, berries, yams, potatoes, broccoli, and legumes.

Having a fiber with every meal works for you in two ways. First, it adds volume to the food you're eating, making you feel fuller longer. Second, it decreases the overall glycemic-index rating of a meal by slowing the absorption of nutrients and blood sugar, making for a more evenly paced digestive process.

When adding fiber to your diet, do it slowly to avoid constipation. For example, throw a few raisins in your oatmeal, or add a few extra veggies to your dinner. Slowly increase these amounts each week so you get used to digesting more fiber on a daily basis. Also drink plenty of water to help move things along in the digestive tract.

WATER, WATER EVERYWHERE . . .

. . . especially in your body! Your body is made up of about 60 percent water, a nutrient you must get from the foods you eat and the drinks you ingest. Water is so essential that your body, which can survive for weeks with no food, will perish after only a few days without water. Proper hydration improves endocrine and liver function, decreases appetite, regulates body temperature, and rids your cells of toxins and wastes. In terms of fat loss, water helps you feel more full and aids in the metabolism of food, extracting nutrients from the meals you eat and more efficiently transporting them to cells.

The human body naturally loses about two quarts of water a day through perspiring, breathing, urinating, and other bodily functions. This water must be replaced to ensure proper hydration and bodily function. If it were up to me,

everyone would drink a gallon of water every day! However, I realize this is a tall order, so I encourage you to drink *at least* a half gallon a day of pure, clean water—not juice or soda or sports drinks—just plain water. Before a workout, have 8–10 ounces of water, and during your session, sip

FIBER IN A NUTSHELL

FIBER BASICS
- Regulates blood sugar
- Comes in two types: soluble and insoluble
- Insoluble fiber promotes regularity
- Soluble fiber helps remove excess cholesterol
- Prevents certain cancers (colon, rectal, prostate)
- Controls hunger and regulates weight

TEN GREAT SOURCES OF FIBER
- beans (black beans, lentils, kidney beans)
- root vegetables (carrots, turnips)
- green leafy vegetables (spinach, cauliflower, broccoli)
- raw nuts and seeds (cashews, peanuts, walnuts, sunflower seeds, flaxseeds)
- seaweed
- dried fruit (raisins, prunes, cranberries)
- whole raw fruits (unpeeled apples, pears, and peaches, bananas, oranges)
- whole grains (wheat, rice, corn, oats)
- whole-grain cereal and bread
- sweet potatoes and yams

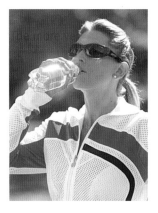

Water Warning!
Don't rely on thirst to tell you when to drink water. By that time, it's usually too late, and you're on your way to becoming dehydrated. Instead, sip water frequently all day long.

Fun Fact
Even mild dehydration can slow the metabolism by up to 3 percent!

WATER IN A NUTSHELL

WATER BASICS
- Cushions bones, organs, and joints
- Regulates body temperature
- Composes about 60 percent of the human body
- Helps metabolize food
- Regulates waste removal
- Decreases appetite
- Decreases bloating

DRINK MORE WATER IF
you're exercising in a hot, humid environment;
you're feeling hungry;
your mouth is dry and sticky;
you're exercising at a higher intensity than normal;
you're exercising longer than normal;
you've had one or more caffeinated beverages;
you've been working or playing outdoors.

TO SPICE UP PLAIN WATER, TRY
- Crystal Light
- a splash of low-sugar fruit juice such as cranberry, apple, grape, or orange
- a twist of mint
- a squeeze of orange, lemon, or lime
- a packet of Real Lemon
- a packet of Emergen-C
- decaf iced tea mix

DID YOU KNOW THAT . . .
drinking water helps alleviate water retention and bloating? Water helps flush out sodium and other bloat-causing elements, so even though it sounds backward, the more water you drink, the less you will retain—trust me!

thirst is often interpreted as hunger? Some people have trouble differentiating between being thirsty and being hungry. If you're feeling some off-hour hunger pangs, slug down a few big glasses of water and see whether they go away.

water frequently. Afterward, drink at least 10–16 ounces of water to replenish what was lost during exercise through sweat, heavy breathing, and cellular reactions.

There are many drinks that can further dehydration rather than relieve it. Coffee, tea, and some sodas contain caffeine, which acts as a diuretic in your body, encouraging cells to release their water and increasing the rate of urination. My rule of thumb is for every caffeinated beverage you have, drink at least twice that much water afterward to account for what you'll be eliminating from the caffeine.

BURNING QUESTION
What's the deal with sports drinks? Sports drinks such as Gatorade and Powerade were designed for use by athletes participating in long, strenuous competitions who needed to replace water, electrolytes, sugars, and salts lost during their sport. However, according to market research, the largest segment of the sports-drink-buying population today is nonathletes! Everywhere I look, I see kids and adults slugging down huge bottles of the stuff with lunch or as a snack. Most people who drink these products casually think they are doing something good for

their bodies and believe these drinks are "better for them" than sodas. While there is some merit to these drinks for the endurance athlete, for the average Joe, they are simply gut bombs. Twelve ounces of Gatorade contains 28 grams of sugar! That's as many as in a full-size Snickers bar, and at least with the Snickers you're getting 4 grams of protein! My advice: Unless you're a marathon runner or soccer player who is on the field for 2–3 hours at a time, skip the sports drinks. Plain water will do you just fine.

SUGAR AND SWEETS

Ask any dieter on the planet where sweets and treats belong in a weight-loss plan and they'll all say: *Nowhere! You can't have sweets when you're trying to lose weight!* For the most part, they're right; you can't have sweet treats all the time and expect to reach your weight-loss goals. Treats are just that—treats. They are to be eaten sparingly and occasionally. But an occasional indulgence shouldn't completely derail your nutrition program, either mentally or physically. Besides, I don't advocate complete elimination of any food group, sweets included. Because hey, chocolate is a big part of my life! I am sure you can relate. So to see where treats can fit into your plan, you've got to analyze what they are made of.

Most sweets and desserts are high in calories and heavy on carbs and fat. Ice cream, chocolate bars, frozen yogurt, pudding, and other dairy-based treats have some protein in them from milk or nuts, in addition to fat and carbohydrates. Treats such as hard candy, sorbet, donuts, and muffins are pretty much straight, simple carbohydrates. Processed baked goods such as cakes, pies, and cookies contain plenty of carbs, maybe a little protein, and a bunch of trans fat to ensure a longer shelf life.

Of course, no one needs the extra calories that come from sweets and desserts, but you can fit the occasional indulgence into a well-planned nutrition schedule without much fuss. We'll discuss meal planning and cheat meals in detail later, but for now, consider these simple guidelines when opting for a treat:

- **Go for homemade.** Avoid processed baked goods and make your own to avoid those nasty trans fats interfering with your tasty goodness.
- **Choose wisely.** If you do have a treat, make sure it's damn good. Don't waste calories on a chocolate chip cookie or coconut cake that isn't the best darn chocolate chip cookie or coconut cake you've ever had in your life!
- **Substitute sugar for starch.** If you're planning on having a dessert with a

Many companies make low-sugar condiments! Check your local grocery store and try some out. They often taste as good as or better than their sugar-full counterparts!

Fast Forward
For more great dessert and treat ideas, turn to page 237!

meal, skip the starch in your entrée, such as potatoes, bread, or pasta, to accommodate the extra calories. Instead, have steamed veggies or a side salad.

- **Learn to share.** One dessert divided six ways at the dinner table will be far less detrimental to your diet than one you eat all yourself!
- **Shrug off the guilt.** If you do have a dessert or sweet treat, eat it slowly and relish the flavor. Good food is a part of life—enjoy it!

Hidden Sugar

Dessert isn't the only place you'll find a ton of sugar: Many condiments, sauces, and dips contain added sugar, as well as many breads, cereals, crackers, and dressings! So before you glop on the barbecue sauce or ketchup, read the label carefully to see how many sugar calories you're getting per serving. Of course, sugar will not always be listed as "sugar" on the label. Usually it goes by one of these aliases:

- maltodextrose
- dextrose
- sucrose
- fructose
- high-fructose corn syrup
- malt syrup
- corn syrup

BURNING QUESTION

What do I do about cravings? There isn't a woman alive who hasn't been ready to kill for a cupcake during that time of the month! Here are some tips on handling cravings:

- *Wait it out.* Sometimes cravings are emotionally driven, and you may be eating sweets in reaction to an event. Before you dig into the donut box, stop, recognize

your craving, and wait to see whether you can deduce its source.

- *Revisit your food journal.* Sometimes sugar cravings are caused by the lack of a certain nutrient in your diet. Look through your food journal to make sure you've been getting enough of all the food groups, making adjustments where necessary.
- *Eat more frequently.* You might crave sugar if you haven't eaten in a long while and your blood sugar is low. Your body knows the fastest way to get its blood sugar back up is to get some simple carbs in there, so it tells you to crave sugar—and you do! Space your meals out more evenly to avoid these sugar crashes.
- *Break the habit.* If you always have dessert with dinner or get a treat every day from the vending machine at 4 p.m., recognize that pattern—then break it! Do something completely different, such as taking a walk or calling a friend instead of hitting the vending machine.
- *Give in!* If your craving is truly PMS related, go ahead and have a treat—just make it a small one. A little goes a long way, and sometimes a piece of hard candy will satisfy your craving for sweets just as well as a whopping piece of cake. My favorite tiny treat is a Halloween-size bag of M&Ms. My treat begins and ends with that little bag!

"FREE" FOODS

I am a big fan of "alternative" food products, because many of them really do help you maintain a low-calorie diet. But it's important to be able to discern what you're getting when you buy these products.

Many manufacturers have come up with fat-free or reduced-fat products to replace their original full-fat items. But know this: Just because it's fat free does not mean it's calorie free! In fact, it's just the opposite. To make up for the lack of flavor and texture when the fat is removed from a product, manufacturers typically add in more sugar and carbs. Sometimes a fat-free or reduced-fat product will have just as many calories as the regular alternative! So before you buy something you think is better for you, check the nutrition label to see whether there really is a difference. If there isn't, heck, go with the real thing! Just have it in moderation.

In sugar-free items, sugar (sucrose) has been replaced by either a sugar alcohol (sorbitol, maltitol, xylitol, mannitol) or a synthetic product (saccharin, NutraSweet). Sugar alcohols are not technically sugar, but they still contain calories from carbohydrates and are not calorie free. The alcohol in these sweeteners attracts water into the gut and can cause abdominal discomfort, bloating, and diarrhea in many people (me included!). Foods sweetened with synthetic products are the ones I recommend if you're gonna go the fake-food route, especially those made with Splenda, which is actually made from sugar. They are typically lower in calories and taste just as good as any full-sugar item out there. But also beware: Just because an item is sugar free does not mean it's fat free! Again, look at the labels carefully to see exactly what you're getting.

ALCOHOL

Invariably, clients ask me where alcohol lands in terms of nutrient profile. That's a tough one because it doesn't fit neatly anywhere. Alcohol is in a category all its own, and while it's often touted as low carb or carb free, it's far from low calorie. Alcohol begins its life as a carbohydrate but turns

Terminology Breakdown

Term	Fat Breakdown
Fat free	Less than 0.5 grams of fat
Low fat	3 grams or less of fat
Reduced (or less) fat	25 percent less fat (than a standard serving of the original food)
Light	A third fewer calories or 50 percent less fat (than a standard serving of the original food)

FREE FOODS IN A NUTSHELL

- Are not necessarily lower in calories
- Might cause digestive distress
- Sugar-free foods contain sugar alcohol or synthetic sugar instead of sucrose (table sugar).
- Fat-free foods often replace fat with sugar and carbs.

into alcohol when microorganisms digest these carbs in the absence of oxygen in a process called fermentation. One gram of alcohol contains 7 calories—that's more than a gram of protein or carbs (4 calories per gram) and almost as many as a gram of fat (9 calories per gram). And for all those calories you get zero (zip, nada, nil) vitamins, minerals, or nutrients at all.

Like everything, alcohol in excess can be fattening: It contains tons of calories, and, even worse, it slows your metabolism! When you have a cocktail, a shot, or a glass of wine, the alcohol in your drink is absorbed directly into the blood from the stomach and small intestines. Here is the

Fun Fact
Fruit makes a great dessert—and it is always fat free! Try fresh pears or apples with a little cinnamon and Splenda!

Booze by the Numbers

Alcohol Serving	Nutrition Breakdown
1.5-ounce shot of 80-proof alcohol	100 calories, 0 grams of carbs
1.5-ounce shot of 100-proof alcohol	124 calories, 0 grams of carbs
6-ounce glass of wine (red)	128 calories, 1.4 grams of carbs
6-ounce glass of wine (white)	120 calories, 3 grams of carbs
6-ounce glass dessert wine (Riesling)	270 calories, 21 grams of carbs
6-ounce glass of port wine	277 calories, 15 grams of carbs
Regular 12-ounce beer (Budweiser)	145 cal, 10.6 grams of carbs
Light 12-ounce beer: (Bud Light)	110 cal, 6.6 grams of carbs
Low-carb 12-ounce beer (Bud Select)	99 cal, 3.1 grams of carbs

ALCOHOL IN A NUTSHELL

- Is metabolized by the liver
- Contains 7 calories per gram
- Is perceived by the liver as toxic
- Contains no vitamins, minerals, or nutrients
- Is absorbed directly into the bloodstream
- Is high in empty calories

kicker, though: The liver is responsible for metabolizing this alcohol, but it's also responsible for metabolizing fats. When you drink, the liver puts the order to digest fats on hold to deal with the alcohol, which it sees as a poison. Therefore, whatever you've been eating is more likely to be stored as fat. Not good when you're trying to lose weight!

There are ways to minimize the impact alcohol has on your diet. If you're going to indulge, consider these suggestions:

- **Be a wine-o.** Not only is wine lower in calories per serving than beer or mixed drinks; research indicates that red wine has antioxidant properties.
- **Sub the soda.** Use diet soda, diet tonic water, or seltzer instead of sugary mixers such as juice, regular soda, and syrup in mixed drinks, and save up to 100 calories per cocktail!

- **Hydrate well.** For every alcoholic drink you have, drink at least one full glass of water. This will help the body metabolize the alcohol and will counteract some of the dehydrating effects of the alcohol on the body (such as next-day hangovers!).
- **Space it out.** It takes your liver 1 hour to process and metabolize 1 ounce of alcohol, so space your drinks out accordingly. The less you overload the liver, the better it will be able to process the alcohol and address any fats waiting to be broken down.
- **Go light.** Choose light beer instead of regular and save up to 50 calories per serving!
- **Consider alcohol a carb.** If you're going to have a drink (or two!) with a meal, cut back on or eliminate the carbs you have with your entrée.
- **Pass on post-meal drinks.** Dessert wine, port, and liqueurs have tons of alcohol and tons of sugar, so skip these or sip them sparingly.

BURNING QUESTION

Are low-carb beers really low carb? Yes, but it varies greatly from brand to brand. Most low-carb beers contain 95–110 calories and between 2.6 and 6.6 grams of carbs per 12-ounce serving. Regular beers, on average, contain 145 calories and 11 grams of carbs per 12-ounce serving. Some light beers, such as Amstel Light, have 95 calories and as few as 5 grams of carbs per serving, which is lower than some advertised low-carb beers out there! If you're concerned about how many carbs your beer has, do some research online and investigate your options. Also do a taste test, because according to most beer drinkers I know, many low-carb beers taste pretty bad. And remember: Low-carb beer is still not low calorie! At 100 or more calories per serving, it adds up quickly, carbs or no carbs.

SODIUM

Sodium, aka salt, is found in nearly all foods but is abundant in processed items, fast foods, and restaurant dishes. Why? Because we're so conditioned to the taste of salt in food that when it does not contain high amounts of sodium, we think the food is boring or bland. The body needs some sodium to regulate fluid balance, transmit nerve impulses, and help the muscles contract and relax, but if we never added a pinch of salt to any of our meals, we'd still get plenty of sodium naturally from our foods. For example, milk, yogurt, beets, eggs, and

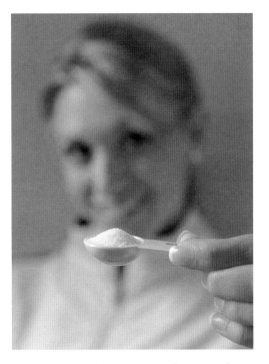

1 teaspoon of salt = 2,400 milligrams of sodium

SODIUM IN A NUTSHELL

SODIUM BASICS

- Regulates fluid balance, transmits nerve impulses, and controls the contraction of muscles
- Is found naturally in many foods
- Is found in abundance in processed and restaurant foods
- Can cause high blood pressure when ingested in excess
- The AHA recommends no more than 2,400 milligrams per day for adults

TEN NOTORIOUS HIGH-SODIUM FOODS

- canned soup
- frozen dinners
- processed lunch meats (salami, bologna, turkey, ham)
- condiments (ketchup, soy sauce, salsa, Worcestershire sauce)
- olives
- pickles
- fast food
- chips, pretzels, popcorn
- canned (versus frozen or fresh) veggies
- salad dressing

SODIUM ALIASES

- monosodium glutamate (MSG)
- sodium nitrite
- sodium saccharin
- baking soda (sodium bicarbonate)
- sodium benzoate
- baking powder
- disodium phosphate
- sodium alginate

SHAKE THE HABIT!

Try these herbs and spices instead of salt:

- *On meats such as beef, lamb, and pork:* bay leaf, marjoram, garlic, rosemary, onion powder, pepper, sage, curry, salt substitute
- *On poultry such as chicken and turkey:* oregano, paprika, rosemary, tarragon, thyme, pepper
- *On fish such as salmon, swordfish, and cod:* bay leaf, dill, mustard, marjoram, cayenne pepper, lemon, paprika, light salt

celery contain a lot of sodium, as do fish, turnips, and artichokes.

According to the American Heart Association, adults should have no more than 2,400 milligrams of sodium per day. Personally, I think that's on the high side, so I recommend between 1,500 and 2,000 milligrams of sodium per day for my clients, with an absolute max of 2,400 milligrams on rare occasions. Because remember: The higher your salt intake, the higher your blood pressure, and the higher your blood pressure, the greater your risk for heart disease, stroke, congestive heart failure, edema, and kidney disease.

BURNING QUESTION

How does sodium cause high blood pressure? Your kidneys regulate the amount of sodium you've got in your body, conserving it when it's scarce and eliminating it when it's abundant. But when the levels are overwhelming, your kidneys can't eliminate it fast enough and it starts to accumulate in your blood. Sodium attracts and holds water, and as a result your blood volume increases. This, in turn, makes your heart work harder to move this higher volume of blood through your vessels, increasing the pressure in your arteries.

SUMMARY

Now you've got a handle on anything and everything nutrition! With your knowledge of protein, carbs, and fat, and your new understanding of fiber, water, alcohol, sugar, sodium, and "free" foods, you're sure to succeed at any and all dietary goals you intend to reach!

HOMEWORK

1. Add more fiber to your diet starting now! Toss a few raisins into your oatmeal, add some chopped veggies to your morning egg whites, or switch from baked potatoes to yams.

2. Fill a gallon container with water. Use this container to pour yourself water all through the day. At the end of the day, see how much water is gone from the container and mark that level with indelible pen. The next day, refill the container and try to outdrink your previous day's level. Continue this process until you can finish off a whole gallon in a day!

3. Read the ingredient labels on all your condiments, sauces, and canned goods, and look at the sodium content. See where you can cut out unnecessary sodium from meals and snacks.

4. Today and the rest of this week, each time you feel a sugar craving, have a piece of peppermint gum instead of chocolate chip cookies or pastry. See what happens! Note your experience and feelings in your food journal.

CHAPTER 14

The Deal with Meals

Fast Forward
Turn to page 255 for tips on dining out healthfully!

The other night, I went to a fancy steak restaurant with my husband for a special occasion. We ordered a steak apiece and two sides to share. When our meals came, holy cow—literally! The steaks were enormous, at least 16 ounces each, and the sides could have comfortably fed a table of six. If I had eaten my whole meal—half of each side and my entire steak—it would have come out to about 4,000 calories—that's 2,300 calories more than I typically eat in a whole day! Of course, I knew better than to eat my whole plate of food, but many people don't realize that portions like this are too big. So in this chapter we are going to address portion control.

PROPER PORTIONS

What exactly is a proper portion of food? That's the million-dollar question and the largest point of confusion with everyone I talk to. With restaurants giving you huge plates of food and fast-food joints encouraging you to supersize everything

(including your butt!), it's easy to get confused. But really, portion control is not rocket science, and I am not going to turn it into rocket science for the sake of selling books. Common sense and a little knowledge can dictate most of your food choices, because really, it's no mystery that snack cakes and French fries are not good for you, or that a burrito as big as your head is too much food at once.

To help you understand proper portion sizes, I've broken it down again into the macronutrients—protein, carbs, and fats.

Protein

Your protein portion should be about the size of a deck of cards in length and width.

A card-size protein portion might not seem like a lot of food to you at first, but this is the amount of protein your body can digest and assimilate at one time. If you ingest more than this, it is more likely to be stored as fat. Remember that any excess calories can be stored as fat, whether they come from carbs, fats, or proteins!

PERFECT PORTIONS

PERFECT PROTEIN PORTION

- 4–5 egg whites
- 1 small skinless chicken breast
- 1 petite filet (4 ounces)
- 1 medium ground-turkey patty
- 1 medium pork chop

PERFECT FAT PORTION

- 1 tablespoon of olive oil
- ¼ avocado
- 10–15 raw almonds
- 1 pat of butter
- 1 tablespoon of peanut butter

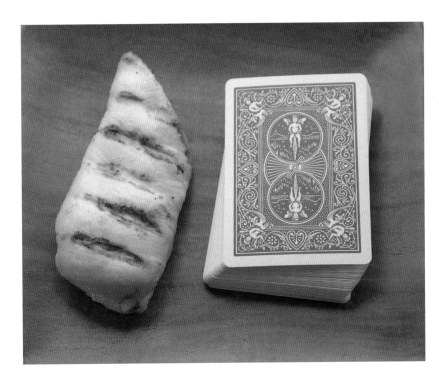

Your protein for each meal should be about the size of a deck of cards in length and width.

Fats

Each meal should contain a serving of fat, which is equal to a golf-ball-size slice of avocado or a tablespoon of peanut butter.

Remember that fats contain a lot of calories per gram, so they should be added sparingly to meals and snacks.

Carbohydrates

Your higher-GI (starchy) carbohydrates, such as fruit, potatoes, whole-wheat bread, or rice, should be about the size of a baseball (not a softball!), or about 1 cup in volume.

This represents the correct amount needed to fuel your metabolism and your

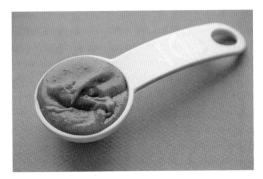

One tablespoon of peanut butter is a perfect serving of fat for one meal.

Food Fact

Be aware of how much fat your protein contains. If you're having a fatty protein such as salmon, herring, or 96 percent fat-free ground beef, you won't need to add any extra fat to your meal.

Food Fact

The more veggies (and fiber) you eat, the longer you'll feel full and the more slowly you'll digest your meal.

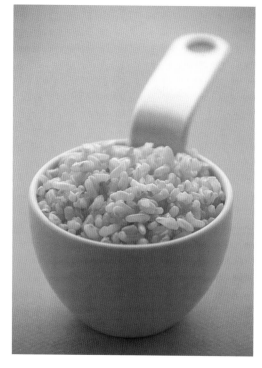

One cup of cooked brown rice is the right amount of carbohydrate for one meal.

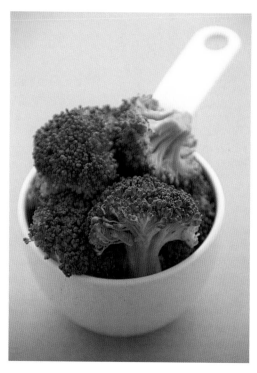

Have at least 1 cup of veggies per meal!

PERFECT PORTIONS

PERFECT CARBOHYDRATE PORTIONS
- 1 cup of brown rice (cooked)
- 1 medium apple
- 1 slice of whole-wheat bread
- 20 grapes
- ½ cup dry oatmeal

PERFECT VEGGIE PORTIONS
- 1 cup of broccoli
- 2 cups of salad greens
- 2 cups of spinach, raw
- 1 cup of asparagus
- 1 cup of carrots

workouts. I recommend you take in the majority of your high-glycemic carbs before 3 p.m. so they go toward that purpose instead of being stored as body fat.

After 3 p.m. I recommend switching from high-glycemic to low-glycemic carbs. Because vegetables are low in calories, you can have a higher volume of them than you can of high-glycemic choices.

Note: Although serving size is crucial to your success, if you're going to go overboard in one direction, do it in the veggie category. The calories are significantly lower and the volume and bulk much higher.

TIMING IS EVERYTHING

With the *Your Body, Your Life* nutrition plan, your daily calories will be broken down into three meals and two snacks daily. Each meal should contain a good balance of protein, carbs, and fat in the portions recommended above. The snacks should contain half as much of each element but should still be balanced and nutritious.

If you're doing the math here, you realize you'll be eating something every 3 to 4 hours, which might sound like a lot at first, but believe me, once your metabolism starts kicking in, you'll be hungry for that next meal or snack! Think of your body as a fireplace. If you throw a log on a hot fire, it will burn quickly. If you let the fire cool, that same log will take twice as long to burn or might not burn completely at all! It's the same with your body: If you give a fired-up metabolism some food, it gets processed and burned quickly. If your metabolism is lukewarm or cold, that same food will break down slowly or even get stored as fat.

By spreading your calories out evenly throughout the day, you'll never have a "crash," where you feel tired, hungry, and crabby because of low blood sugar. Your metabolism will remain active, running in high gear all day long, burning more calories and increasing your weight-loss potential.

The prospect of eating five times a day may sound daunting to many of you, but it's not as hard as you might think. Yes, it will take some planning and foresight on your part, but this planning will get much easier and will become second nature in no time.

Let's look at Brenda's meal schedule, for example. Brenda gets up at 7 a.m. to get to work by 8:30 a.m. She works out in the evenings at 5:30 p.m.

7 a.m.:	breakfast (meal 1)
10 a.m.:	snack 1
1 p.m.:	lunch (meal 2)
4 p.m.:	snack 2
5:30 p.m.:	workout
7 p.m.:	dinner (meal 3)

Notice that there is never more than a 3-hour gap between Brenda's meals. This guarantees that Brenda will never get to the point where she feels like she is starving and crams a donut in her mouth in desperation. She will feel energetic and satisfied all day long with this schedule and will be able to fuel her metabolism and her workout properly.

Now let's look at Donna's meal schedule, which is slightly different from Brenda's. Donna works out in the morning before her job and gets to work by 9:30 a.m.

5:30 a.m.:	snack 1
6 a.m.:	workout
8 a.m.:	breakfast (meal 1)
12 p.m.:	lunch (meal 2)
3 p.m.:	snack 2
7 p.m.:	dinner (meal 3)

Donna has adjusted her schedule a bit to accommodate her needs. She doesn't like to work out on an empty stomach, so she eats one of her snacks first thing in the morning. Then, after her workout, she has breakfast as her first full meal. Even though she has shuffled things around a bit, Donna still has something to eat every 3 to 4 hours and will keep her metabolism going all day long.

Many people ask me, "Can't I just eat two big meals a day instead of five?" The short answer: No! Your body can handle and metabolize only about 400–500 calories at a time; anything eaten above and beyond that number is going to be put away in storage for later use as body fat. Why? Because when you eat a very large meal, you flood your body with calories, causing a huge spike in blood sugar. Your body produces a ton of insulin to keep up with the food breakdown, and mops up a ton of glucose. Some of the glucose goes to fuel the metabolism, but the extra calories you've taken in will be stored as fat.

Food Fact
When you "crash," you're more likely to grab fast, sugary carbs such as a minimuffin or a handful of chips to quickly elevate your blood sugar.

To avoid storing unnecessary fat, give your body smaller amounts of calories more frequently throughout the day. That way the body can break the food down, assimilate it, and use it. By the time it's done with one batch of calories, in comes another one! The metabolism fires back up again and the process starts over.

BURNING QUESTION

Do I have to eat breakfast? Yes, yes, and to reiterate—*yes*! Many people still think that the easiest way to lose weight is by skipping meals, and the meal people most commonly skip is breakfast. This drives me crazy because—your mom was right!—this really is the most important meal of the day. Think about it: You've literally been fasting since dinnertime at 7 p.m. the night before. If you don't "break" your "fast" by eating a meal in the morning at 7 a.m., and hold out on food until lunch at noon, you're asking your body to go a grand total of 17 hours without food! *Screeeeech*! That was your metabolism hitting the brakes. Just eat breakfast, people! And the excuse *I don't have time for breakfast* does not fly with me. It only takes minutes to nuke some egg whites or boil water for oatmeal. This is how easy breakfast can be:

- *Easy Eggs:* 5 microwaved egg whites with 1 slice whole-wheat toast and 1 slice low-fat cheese
- *Protein Smoothie:* 1 scoop whey protein powder with 1 cup nonfat milk and 1 teaspoon almond butter
- *Super Oatmeal:* ½ cup dry instant oatmeal with ½ cup skim milk and 1 tablespoon peanut butter.

See? No more excuses! Just set your alarm 5 minutes earlier (and stop hitting that snooze button!) and you'll have plenty of time for breakfast.

CALORIE CRAZY

Unlike many trainers, I am not obsessive about counting calories. You should be familiar with the approximate calorie counts for your meals and snacks, but don't nitpick and count every little thing— you'll go crazy! I know I told you in Chapter 5 to write down everything you put into your mouth in your food journal, and I stand by that exercise as a great way to help you get real about what you're actually eating. I also still believe in keeping a food journal as a way to keep track of your nutrition over the long term and help identify patterns of emotional eating. But honestly, at the end of the day, if you've gone over or under your daily target by 100–200 calories, it's not the end of the world! It's just life. If you give yourself overly stringent guidelines and miss your mark a few times, you'll be more likely to begin a pattern of self-denial, punishment, and restriction, which many times can be as unhealthy as bingeing and can also lead to destructive relationships with food.

To keep everyone sane, I suggest setting up a "ballpark" range of between 1,200 and 1,700 calories a day. If you're not sure where to start, begin with about 1,500 calories and go up or down from there. There is no exact science or elaborate mathematical equation to these numbers; it's more a matter of common sense. If you're having a particularly active day, eat a little bit more. If you're having a sedentary day, eat less! Besides, it's good to change your caloric intake slightly from day to day. If you eat 1,200 calories every day, your body will get used to that number and will begin to use that fuel more efficiently, meaning you'll have a harder time losing weight. So plan on having some days with higher calories and others with lower calories to keep the body guessing and your weight loss progressing.

Remember you've got to break your daily calories down into three meals and two snacks a day. Let's take 1,500 calories a day, for example. You could break that evenly into 400 calories for each meal and 150 calories for each snack. Or you could have one meal of 500 calories, two meals of 325, one snack of 200, and one of 150. Nothing is set in stone. Play with your calorie splits and see what works best for you in terms of energy maintenance and work and exercise schedules.

BURNING QUESTION

What is a calorie? Calories are simply a measure of how much energy a food provides your body when it's consumed. The more calories a food contains, the more potential energy it supplies your body. The number of calories your body requires to be alive and function on a daily basis is called your basal metabolic rate (BMR). This includes the number of calories it takes to think, digest, breathe, type, sit, shower, and even eat! All these actions require energy. As we discussed in Chapter 2, your BMR is affected by your individual age, height, gender, activity level, body composition (fat weight versus muscle weight), and diet. The more active you are, the higher your BMR will be.

UNDEREATING

Have you ever been on a diet where you ate close to nothing and weren't losing any weight? Many people have had this experience, and this is a really common complaint for chronic calorie-cutting dieters. If you cut calories time and again over the years in a vain effort to lose weight, oftentimes you end up eating fewer than 1,000 calories a day! In reaction, your body becomes more efficient with a lower caloric intake and burns fewer calories than it did previously, essentially shutting off your metabolism and putting your body in starvation, or survival, mode. In this survival mode, your body will store any calories taken in as fat instead of burning them off, even supposedly "good" calories that come from fruit or healthy carbs. The body does not differentiate when it thinks it's starving—everything goes into storage to protect the internal organs. Remember, too, that in this state, the body uses muscle tissue as fuel instead of fat, furthering the metabolic shutdown. To keep your metabolism going, you've got to keep your basal metabolic rate high. To do that, you've got to supply it with enough calories to run the body efficiently, at least 1,200–1,700 daily.

SAMPLE CALORIE SCHEDULES

Let's go one step further and see how these three meals and two snacks might break down into an actual menu plan. Using some of the recipes from Chapter 16 as well as some common healthy foods, I have put together three sample meal plans for you to check out. Remember—these plans are here only to give you an idea of how to break things down! These are not by any means a strict eating plan for you to follow. You can certainly use them if you'd like, but, heck, you might hate chicken or be allergic to strawberries! Use these as guidelines to formulate your own plans that fit your tastes and lifestyle.

Web Watch
To accurately calculate the calorie content of a meal, snack, or food item, go to www.calorieking.com. I used this site for all the recipes in Chapter 16, as well as when formulating meal plans for clients on television and off.

1,300 Calories

Breakfast	Snack	Lunch	Snack	Dinner
1 tall Starbucks nonfat latte, 4 egg whites, Maple-Meal Oatmeal (page 224)	1 slice whole-grain toast, 1 Dannon Light & Fit Smoothie	Personal Pizza (page 228)	PB & A (page 223)	Grilled Halibut Amandine (page 234), Roasted Asparagus (page 232), Chocolate-Dipped Cherries (page 224)

Breakdown: calories 1,306; fat 36 grams; carbs 158 grams; protein 101 grams, fiber 22 grams

1,500 Calories

Breakfast	Snack	Lunch	Snack	Dinner
1 cup green tea, 1 Morningstar Farms Veggie Breakfast Sausage Patty, 4 egg whites, 1 slice whole wheat toast	2 tablespoons peanut butter, 2 rice cakes, 1 banana	1 grilled chicken breast (4–6 ounces), 1 serving (½ cup) Spanish rice (page 233), 1 sugar-free Popsicle	1 small no-sugar-added vanilla latte (Coffee Bean and Tea Leaf), 1 Magic Muffin (page 225)	1 serving Turkey Meatloaf (page 233), mixed grilled veggies

Breakdown: calories 1,508; fat 38 grams; carbs 157 grams; protein 141 grams; fiber 19 grams

1,700 Calories

Breakfast	Snack	Lunch	Snack	Dinner
Berri-licious Crepes (page 225), ½ cup light OJ	1 piece low-fat string cheese, 22 raw unsalted almonds	1 chicken breast, 1 cup brown rice, 1 cup broccoli	Wasa Bruschetta (page 224)	Excellent Enchiladas (page 236), small green salad with 10 squirts Wish-Bone Salad Spritzer, Banana Split Crunch (page 237)

Breakdown: calories 1,717; fat 36 grams; carbs 190 grams; protein 100 grams; fiber 22 grams

CHEAT MEALS

I am a huge believer in cheat meals, because, as you know, sometimes you just *have* to have a pizza or a slice of cheesecake! And believe it or not, eating your "vice" foods once in a while can be beneficial. It will alleviate any desperate cravings you're having, making it more likely you'll stick to your diet over the long term. It will also throw your body a curveball—just when your body is becoming more efficient at using the foods you've been eating consistently, you douse it with eggs benedict or an ice cream sundae! Your body forgets all it had learned about your eating patterns and "resets" its gears. Many times, when people are stuck on a plateau, all they need to get themselves rolling again is a good cheat meal.

The trick with cheat meals, however, is control! It's a cheat *meal*, people, not a cheat day or a cheat week. Limit your cheating to one single meal and don't go completely overboard. For that meal, have whatever you've been craving, be it a cheeseburger with fries and a shake, or pasta Alfredo, a glass of wine, and tiramisu for dessert. Eat your meal slowly, enjoy every bite, and shrug off any guilt lurking in the background. This meal is necessary to your mental and physical well-being, so savor it—then get right back to healthy eating!

SUMMARY

So you've finally discovered the true secret to weight loss: portion control and meal planning! If you take your new knowledge of nutrition from Chapters 12 and 13, and apply it to what you learned in this chapter, you'll be well on your way to losing weight and keeping it off.

HOMEWORK

1. Go to a restaurant and order a regular entrée. Use the dining-out guidelines to pare your meal down to an appropriate portion.
2. Sit down with your weekly schedule. Plan when you're going to eat each of your three meals and two snacks.
3. Write out a meal and snack schedule of your own using the recipes from Chapter 16 or common foods you plan on eating for 1,300, 1,500, and 1,700 calories.
4. Today and the rest of this week, take your lunch and snacks with you in a small cooler to work or while running errands.

Extra Credit

Go to my Web site (www.kimlyons.com), and click on "BMR Calculator." Enter a few simple numbers and figure out your BMR, the absolute baseline number of calories you need to keep your body alive.

CLIENT CORNER

ALL OR NOTHING, BY KAI

I have an all-or-nothing mentality and struggle with the idea that it's OK to have a brownie now and then, but that it's not OK to eat the whole pan—and then cry about it! I am one of those people who think, *I had a sugar cookie and blew my diet; I might as well eat a bucket of fried chicken for dinner and follow that up with a whole cheesecake!* For that reason, I never, ever ate the foods I was craving when I was trying to lose weight. But eventually, I hit a big plateau in my progress. I was so frustrated! Kim and I reviewed my journals and agreed that I should moderate my activity for a while since it was obvious I was overtraining, but when she tried to get me to have a cheat meal as a break from my diet, I refused! I was scared I would not be able to control myself, that I would stuff my face with the foods I used to love, and that I would pork back up to 262 pounds! I finally relented and did it—and I was surprised: I could control myself and limit my cheating to just one meal! Once I had eaten it, I felt guilty, but eventually I learned that it would not make me blow back up again to have a cheeseburger every once in a while.

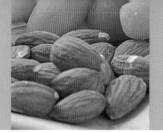

CHAPTER 15

Grocery Shopping and Meal Planning

Food for Thought
If your tempting food or product is unopened, don't eat it! Instead, consider donating it to a food bank or homeless shelter instead of throwing it away!

It's time to go shopping! As any good shopper knows, when you buy something new, you've got to get rid of something old. In this case, you'll be cleansing your kitchen of everything unhealthy or tempting and replacing it with all things healthy and wholesome! If it's not in your house, you won't eat it! This may even be a very cathartic process, because you are literally tossing out your old way of life to make way for a new one. So scour your cabinets and throw away these things:

- full-fat cheese, milk, and other dairy products
- full-fat salad dressings, mayonnaise, and other fatty condiments
- high-sodium sauces, soups, or condiments
- processed snack foods such as crackers, chips, cookies, and granola bars
- sugary cereals
- ice cream and high-sugar frozen yogurt
- frozen dinners, Lunchables, or other prepackaged, processed meals

- high-sodium, high-fat lunch meat, sausage, and hot dogs
- bacon, spare ribs
- high-fat ground beef, turkey, or chicken
- white flour, white sugar, white rice, and white bread

BURNING QUESTION

My kids like sugary snacks and chips as after-school treats—should I throw them away, too? It's a good idea to get rid of tempting foods, but don't toss out all your kids' favorite foods without an explanation. You'll have family anarchy! Instead, sit down with your family and explain that you are trying to get healthy and lose weight, and that you need to limit the amount of unhealthy foods in the house so you're not tempted to eat them. Usually you have to tell your kids your intentions only once, and all of a sudden you've got a bunch of little food Nazis running around reminding you not to eat bad things! One technique that works well is giving your

kids the lowest shelf in the snack cabinet—
the one you can't reach without really
trying, or see without bending down—for
their treats and snacks. When you go
shopping, allow them to choose two snack
foods, sugary treats, or cereals per week,
and put them away in their own special
cabinet. That way, they feel empowered to
make their own food decisions instead
of restricted or deprived. By the by, it's not
a bad idea to try to get your kids to eat
healthier, too, but don't announce you're
going to do it, by any means! That is a
sure-fire way to get them to rebel, insisting
that the food tastes funny or bad. Instead,
quietly swap out full-fat or unhealthy
items for foods such as low-fat mayo,
low-fat cheese, reduced-sugar cereal and
snacks, and whole-wheat bread or
pasta. Chances are they will never know
the difference!

Now that you've purged your kitchen
of anything and everything unhealthy, it's
time to restock it with fabulous food! On
the following pages, you'll find two shopping lists. The first one is the Getting
Started list. These are the foods I want you
to go out and buy right now, pronto, as in
today! The second list is foods to buy in a
few weeks when you've gotten the hang of
the Getting Started foods and are ready to
flex your cooking muscles a bit.

SHOP SMART!

Here are some suggestions to make your grocery store experience
smooth and easy!

- *Meditate on menus.* Before hitting the grocery store, think about
  what you want to cook and how much of it you need to make
  meals for the week. Write out a list of foods that you need for the
  recipes you'll be using.
- *Cut coupons.* Eating healthy isn't always cheap—this is where your
  coupon-cutting skills come in handy! Check your local grocery
  flyers and newspaper ads to see what's on sale. Buy plenty of the
  items you're gunning for in bulk, especially meats and poultry,
  and freeze them for later use.
- *Befriend the butcher.* Your local butcher can do special things for
  you—if you ask him (or her) nicely! Have your butcher grind up
  your skinless chicken breasts into patties to make chicken
  burgers, or ask whether special meat or fish products such as
  grass-fed organic beef or wild salmon steaks are available or can
  be ordered.
- *Avoid autopilot shopping.* There are lots of healthy items to be
  had at your grocery store if you know where to look. "Less popular" healthy products are usually on the extreme lower or upper
  shelves, while the more commonly purchased, heavily advertised
  stuff is in the middle. For example, slow-cooking oatmeal is on the
  bottom shelf of most grocery stores, while Froot Loops is right at
  eye level (or kids' eye level!)

GETTING STARTED SHOPPING LIST
Meats
- boneless, skinless chicken breasts
- salmon
- 99 percent fat-free ground turkey
- chunk-white low-sodium tuna in water

Dairy
- low-fat or fat-free cheeses
- fat-free cottage cheese
- nonfat milk
- I Can't Believe It's Not Butter! spray
- eggs

Fruits and Vegetables
- broccoli
- asparagus
- tomatoes
- cucumbers
- lettuce
- avocado
- onion
- garlic
- sweet potatoes
- green beans
- apples
- strawberries
- lemon

Beans, Rice, and Bread
- black beans
- oatmeal
- brown rice
- whole-wheat bread
- Wasa crackers

Drinks
- green tea (tea bags)
- sparkling water
- coffee

Spices, Dressings, and Condiments
- balsamic vinegar
- fat-free salad dressing
- extra-virgin olive oil
- low-sodium/low-carb ketchup
- yellow or spicy mustard
- nonfat mayonnaise
- Mrs. Dash's spices (all kinds)
- ground pepper

Miscellaneous
- regular or olive oil nonfat cooking spray
- Splenda granular or packets
- light or low-sugar fruit spread or jam
- all-natural or reduced-fat peanut butter
- raw nuts (almonds, cashews, walnuts)
- whole flaxseeds

GENERAL GROCERY LIST
Meat, Chicken, and Fish
- lean or extra-lean ground beef, ground turkey breast, or ground chicken breast
- top sirloin steak
- lean beef filets
- pork tenderloin
- boneless, skinless chicken breasts
- fresh fish (salmon, tuna, halibut, red snapper, sea bass)
- shrimp, fresh or frozen
- low-sodium deli-sliced chicken, ham, turkey, or roast beef
- Canadian bacon or turkey bacon
- chunk-white low-sodium tuna in water

Dairy
- Laughing Cow low-fat cheese triangles
- low- or nonfat cheddar, pepper jack, mozzarella, ricotta, parmesan, or cottage cheese
- nonfat milk
- I Can't Believe It's Not Butter! spray
- eggs
- packaged egg whites or Egg Beaters
- low-fat cheese sticks or string cheese
- Dannon Light & Fit Carb & Sugar Control yogurt
- Cool Whip fat-free whipped topping

Fruits and Vegetables

- broccoli
- green beans
- spaghetti squash
- cauliflower
- asparagus
- carrots
- cucumbers
- bell peppers
- avocado
- celery
- squash
- eggplant
- Brussels sprouts
- zucchini
- mushrooms
- cherry tomatoes
- bags of lettuce (all kinds)
- spinach
- red apples
- Granny Smith apples
- strawberries
- blueberries
- raspberries
- blackberries
- lemons
- yams
- sweet potatoes
- onions
- garlic

Beans, Rice, Cereal, and Bread

- beans* (pinto, black, white, or lima beans; peas; lentils)
- wild rice
- brown rice
- whole-wheat bread
- whole-wheat tortillas
- Wasa crackers
- old-fashioned or instant oatmeal
- Kashi Go Lean cereal
- all-natural bran cereal
- oat bran

*Beans are dried or low-sodium canned.

Drinks

- green tea (tea bags)
- Diet Snapple (any flavor)
- Crystal Light drink mixes
- Hansen's diet soda (any flavor)
- Hansen's low-carb smoothie (any flavor)
- sparkling water
- coffee
- light fruit juices
- no-sugar-added hot cocoa

Spices, Dressings, and Condiments

- balsamic or red wine vinegar
- Wish-Bone Salad Spritzers
- fat-free or light salad dressings
- extra-virgin olive oil
- garlic powder
- Tabasco sauce
- low-sodium/low-carb ketchup
- mustard (yellow, Dijon, or spicy)
- low-carb barbeque sauce
- Mrs. Dash 10-Minute Marinades
- Mrs. Dash spices (all kinds)
- nonfat mayonnaise
- vanilla extract
- low-sodium soy sauce
- kosher salt
- ground pepper
- cinnamon

Miscellaneous

- regular or olive oil nonfat cooking spray
- Splenda (granular and packets)
- light or low-sugar fruit spread or jam
- sugar-free Popsicles
- all-natural or reduced-fat peanut butter
- raw nuts (almonds, cashews, walnuts)
- whole flaxseeds
- ground flaxseed meal
- sugar-free gelatin dessert
- sugar-free pudding

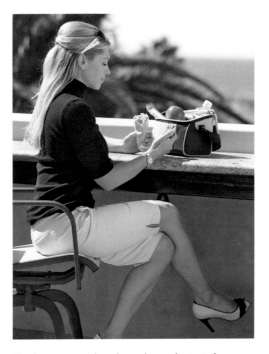

Pack your own lunch and snacks to take to work!

MEAL PLANNING

If you want to succeed with weight loss, you should never leave your nutrition to chance. This is why you should plan for all your meals and snacks ahead of time so you're never at the mercy of the drive-through.

The first thing I recommend is purchasing an inexpensive, portable cooler or soft-sided lunch box, and two refreezable cold packs. The cooler should be big enough to hold at least one meal and two snacks, and the cold packs should last a full day in the cooler. Next, buy a bunch of baggies and plastic containers of varying sizes. (Make sure the containers fit into your new cooler!) This cooler is now your new best friend. Take it with you to work, to your kids' soccer games, to the beach—everywhere you go! Inside your cooler you should pack enough meals and snacks to nourish you for the duration of your time away from your kitchen.

Here are some helpful tips to make planning the meals you put in the cooler, on the breakfast table, and on the dinner table a little easier.

- **Cook in bulk.** Dedicate a few hours every week to cooking up a large batch of protein, such as chicken, fish, or steak, or a bunch of slow-cooking carbs such as yams, sweet potatoes, or brown rice. Parcel out the food into proper portions for the week, freezing some for use later and refrigerating that which you plan on using sooner. You can even pack your protein, carbs, fats, and veggies as complete meals into separate containers so you'll only have to grab a Tupperware and go!
- **Chop, chop.** Once you get your fresh veggies home, chop them up and put them in separate containers or baggies. Store them front and center in your fridge, where they are handy and you won't forget about them! Now it's easy to

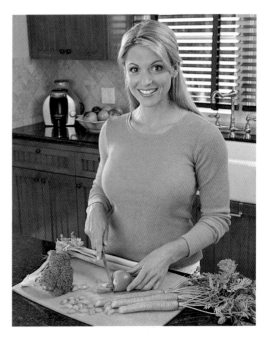

Precut your veggies and fruits so they are ready in a snap!

grab a handful of vegetables and toss them in your morning eggs, or whip together a great dinner salad in no time.

• **Buy prepackaged and precut.** If you legitimately don't have time to cut up a bunch of vegetables or wash and chop a head of lettuce, go for the prepackaged and precut alternatives offered at many grocery stores. These cost a bit more but are handy options for busy people.

• **Make more.** If you're making a recipe such as chili, tacos, soup, or a casserole, make a double batch instead of a single one. These meals will keep for several days in the refrigerator and are great leftovers to be reheated in a pinch for lunch or dinner.

• **Love your leftovers.** Whether you've taken some food home from a restaurant or made extra food the night before, leftovers make great lunches or next-day dinners. Take that grilled chicken and toss it on a salad, or throw it in with some rice and steamed veggies for a rice bowl. Take your extra baked yams, a few raisins, and some cinnamon and Splenda and make a sweet side dish to go with leftover flank steak. Be creative!

• **Make the most of your kitchen time.** While your fish is broiling or your rice is steaming, chop some veggies for an omelet in the morning, make and wrap your sandwich for lunch the next day, or even toss some chicken in to marinate for tomorrow's dinner. You're in the kitchen anyhow—may as well make the most of it!

• **Bother your butcher (again!).** When buying fresh fish, ask the butcher (nicely!) to remove the skin from the fish, and cut it into 4–5 ounce portions. If you're especially nice, your butcher might even wrap each portion separately so there is no question as to whether you're having too much or too little when you cook it up for a meal.

TEN THINGS EVERY HEALTHY KITCHEN SHOULD HAVE

• a sharp knife
• a rice/vegetable steamer
• five different sizes of plastic containers
• nonfat cooking spray
• a plastic or glass cutting board
• five new sponges
• 3 different sizes of baggies (snack, quart, and gallon)
• a blender
• measuring cups and spoons
• 3 nonstick pans

HOW TO READ A FOOD LABEL

It's very important to know how to read a food label. Don't worry—it's not as confusing as you think! In fact, it's relatively simple. You've just got to stop and think a minute or two when deciding on products to purchase or pass on at the store.

First and foremost, look at the calorie content, nutrient breakdown, and sodium content of the product you're considering. See how many calories there are per serving, and how many servings there are per container. Many times people forget to take this step and think they are having 200 calories when really they're having 2,000! (One serving of the item may be 200 calories, but there could be 10 servings per container!) Next, read how many grams of carbs, protein, and fat the product contains per serving to see how it will fit into your nutrition plan overall. Also check whether the product contains any fiber, which lowers the glycemic index (GI) rating of the product, affecting the impact the carbs have on your system. Any sugars in the item also affect the GI rating of the food, moving it up on the GI scale

FOOD-WHIZ

I have made up a mystery product called "Food-Whiz" to demonstrate all the aspects of the nutrition label you'll need to know.

The *serving size* **(A)** for Food-Whiz is 3.5 ounces. However, there are four *servings per container* **(B)**, meaning the entire package contains 14 ounces. The information provided in the Nutrition Facts pertains to only one single serving, one-quarter of the total package.

There are 180 *calories per single serving* **(C)** of Food-Whiz. Since there are four servings to a container, this means that a whole package of Food-Whiz has 720 calories.

A whopping 70 *calories* per single serving of Food-Whiz comes *from fat* **(C)** —nearly a third of the total calories—3 grams of which are *saturated fat* **(D)** calories. Not so good. Fortunately, Food-Whiz does not contain any *trans fats* **(E)**.

Food-Whiz also contains 20 milligrams of *cholesterol* **(F)** per serving, which is of concern to people with high blood pressure and those who are at higher risk for heart disease.

Food-Whiz has 820 milligrams of *sodium* **(G)** for one serving. The whole container, therefore, has a total of 3,280 milligrams of sodium—one and a half times the daily recommended allowance! This is very high.

Food-Whiz has 14 grams of *carbs* **(H)** per serving (56 per container), which is moderate. It also has 3 grams of *fiber* **(I)**, making the impact of these carbs lower on your system and the overall GI rating of the product less than if it had no fiber.

This product only has 1 gram of *sugar* **(J)** per serving, which is not too bad. Remember: The more sugar a product contains, the more refined it is and the faster it will spike your blood sugar.

The *protein* **(K)** content of Food-Whiz is pretty good, coming in at 7 grams per serving, or 28 grams for the whole container. If you ate the whole container, you'd get nearly half of your recommended protein allowance in one sitting.

Overall, Food-Whiz is not a product you should buy on a regular basis (that is, if it were real!). Even though the protein content is high and the fiber is pretty good per serving, Food-Whiz contains a ton of sodium and an unhealthy dose of fat and cholesterol. If you really love Food-Whiz, you can have it occasionally; just limit yourself to one serving at a time and drink a lot of water to counteract the sodium!

NUTRITION FACTS

A — Serving Size 3.5 oz. (28 g)
B — Servings per container 4

Amount Per Serving

C — **Calories** 180	Calories from fat 70

	% Daily Value
Total Fat 7g	11%
D — Saturated Fat 3g	15%
E — *Trans* Fat 0g	
F — **Cholesterol** 20mg	7%
G — **Sodium** 820mg	34%
H — **Total Carbohydrate** 14g	5%
I — Dietary Fiber 3g	14%
J — Sugars 1g	
K — **Protein** 7g	14%

closer to 100 and increasing the calorie content. Finally, see whether the item has any trans fats or cholesterol, which affect your overall health and well-being.

BURNING QUESTION

I bought a "no-sugar-added" product, but there are 4 grams of sugar listed in the Nutrition Facts. What gives? Any product that does not add sugar in the processing or packaging of the food can label it as "no-sugar-added." This does not mean, however, that a product did not already contain sugar before it was processed. Take applesauce, for example. My generic brand of "no-sugar added" applesauce that I just pulled from the cabinet contains 12 grams of sugar per ½-cup serving, and the ingredients are simply apples, water, and ascorbic acid (vitamin C). This is because apples naturally contain sugar. The manufacturer did not add more sugar to the applesauce to make it sweeter, so it can be labeled "no-sugar-added" even though it contains sugar naturally. Overall, a no-sugar-added product will be better for you than one to which sugar has been added. Check it out: The next time you go to the grocery store, look carefully at the applesauce labels. You'll notice a significant difference between the products that add sugar and those that don't.

SUMMARY

Now that you've rid your kitchen and your life of unhealthy foods and filled it with wholesome, fresh ingredients, don't you feel great? Many people love this process and are totally excited to get started on their new, healthy eating plan! I hope you feel this way, too. Stock your home with terrific food, plan your meals carefully, and read food labels diligently, and I know you'll succeed!

HOMEWORK

1. Read the label on your favorite processed-food items. Calculate the calorie content per serving, as well as the macronutrient breakdown, and write them down in your food journal. When you crave these items, open your journal to remind yourself how bad they are for your body!

2. Compare the labels of two similar items in the grocery store (for example, salted roasted almonds versus raw unsalted ones.) Notice the difference across the board in the Nutrition Facts.

3. If you don't have all the items listed in the sidebar "10 Things Every Healthy Kitchen Should Have," go out and buy them today!

4. Sit down and write out a menu of meals for the next few days, then make a grocery list of things you need to buy at the store.

5. Sit down with your schedule and find a few hours when you can cook up a bunch of food for your week.

CHAPTER 16

Kim's Recipes

NOTABLE RECIPE NOTES

- All recipes contain fewer than 4 grams of saturated fat per serving.
- Some recipes are more involved than others but typically make a greater volume of food and can be eaten several times in a week as lunch or dinner.
- Some of the lunch and dinner recipes call for precooked chicken. You can use canned chicken breast, but canned products typically contain a lot of sodium. Instead, I recommend cooking a batch of "neutral" (i.e., unseasoned) chicken once a week that can easily be diced up and added to recipes with no fuss. Boiling whole chicken breasts in water, baking them in the oven, or even dicing and steaming them works great. Store your cooked chicken in an airtight container in the refrigerator and pull it out whenever you're in need.

Have fun with your food! These recipes are not set in stone, and you're free to play with them and add spices and other healthy ingredients to suit your tastes.

I love to cook and experiment with healthy recipes! My friends and family have been my willing guinea pigs over the years, giving the thumbs-up or thumbs-down on my crazy concoctions, and as a result I have come up with a roster of darn good meals and snacks! Now you can garner the benefits of their adventurous taste testing with the *Your Body, Your Life* recipes.

Many times your meals will be as simple as a grilled chicken breast with steamed vegetables and a drizzle of olive oil. But if you want to get creative, this chapter offers some great recipes for breakfast, lunch, dinner, and snacks, as well as a number of desserts and side dishes! The recipes are simple, healthy, and wholesome, and fit nicely into the *Your Body, Your Life* meal plan. Better yet, none of them take more than 30 minutes to prepare! That's faster than the Chinese restaurant takes to deliver, so no more excuses—get in the kitchen and start cooking!

Bon appétit!

SNACKS

Whereas most diet plans tell you snacking is a no-no, I encourage it! "Grazing" throughout the day keeps your metabolism running in high gear and prevents you from overeating at meal time. Sometimes it's tough to come up with a good balanced snack that doesn't blow your daily calories off the chart, so I've put together some snack suggestions that contain protein, carbs, and fat and have between 100 and 250 calories each. These snacks are perfect on the go, at your desk, or at home. In time, you'll come up with your own snack combos that work with your tastes and schedule, but for now, regress to grade school with some Kiddie Stix, or cure your crazy sweet tooth with Chocolate-Dipped Cherries!

Kiddie Stix

    6 celery stalks
    2 tablespoons reduced-fat
        peanut butter

calories 193; fat 12 grams; carbs 15 grams; protein 7 grams; fiber 2 grams

Simply Nuts

    22 whole, dry-roasted almonds

calories 160; fat 15 grams; carbs 5.5 grams; protein 6 grams; fiber 3 grams

Light Fruit and Cheese

    1 medium apple
    1 piece light string cheese

calories 105; fat 3 grams; carbs 15 grams; protein 6 grams; fiber 2.5 grams

PB & A

    1 medium apple
    2 tablespoons reduced-fat
        peanut butter

calories 245; fat 12 grams; carbs 30 grams; protein 7 grams; fiber 5 grams

---

BRIGHT IDEA

Take this PB & A to work! Slice your apple extra thin and place slices in a Ziploc baggie with a squeeze of lemon to keep them from browning. Put your peanut butter into a small plastic container. At snack time, spread a really thin layer of peanut butter on each apple slice, and make this tasty treat last a long time!

Smooth and Nutty

    Dannon Light & Fit Smoothie
    ¼ cup dry-roasted unsalted peanuts

calories 230; fat 17 grams; carbs 9 grams; protein 14 grams; fiber 2 grams

Bright Idea

Higher-sodium recipes are denoted with an asterisk (*).

Rewind

For sample meal plans containing the *Your Body, Your Life* recipes, turn to page 212.

Have a great recipe you'd like to share? E-mail me at www.kimlyons.com!

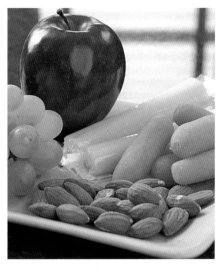

Some of my favorite snack options!

Chocolate-Dipped Cherries (or Strawberries!)

15 pitted cherries
1 container (3.7 ounces) of sugar-free chocolate pudding

Dip cherries in pudding one by one.

calories 124; fat 2 grams; carbs 30 grams; protein 3 grams; fiber 3 grams

Cottage Cheese Crunch

½ cup fat-free cottage cheese
1 tablespoon Smucker's sugar-free jam
½ cup bran cereal

Put ingredients into a small bowl, mix well, and dig in!

calories 140; fat 1 gram; carbs 33 grams; protein 15 grams; fiber 13 grams

Wasa Bruschetta

1 wedge Laughing Cow light cheese
3 Crisp'n Light Wasa crackers
6 slices of tomato
3 teaspoons olive oil

Evenly spread ⅓ of the cheese on each Wasa cracker. Top each cracker with two slices of tomato and drizzle each with a teaspoon of olive oil.

calories 231; fat 16 grams; carbs 18 grams; protein 5 grams; fiber 3 grams

---

BRIGHT IDEA
Sprinkle bruschetta with a tiny bit of garlic salt for extra flavor!

Ham and Cheese Crunch-wich

1 wedge Laughing Cow light cheese
3 Crisp'n Light Wasa crackers
3 thin slices of extra-lean ham

Spread the cheese on the Wasa crackers and top with the ham.

calories 164; fat 4 grams; carbs 15 grams; protein 8 grams; fiber 2 grams

Popcorn Done Right

3 tablespoons unpopped popcorn
I Can't Believe It's Not Butter! spray

Place the popcorn in a paper bag and spray with 5 squirts of I Can't Believe It's Not Butter! spray. Shake the bag, then roll the end tight and microwave for 1–2 minutes or until popping stops.

calories 124; fat 2 grams; carbs 29 grams; protein 4 grams; fiber 6 grams

BREAKFAST

Mom was right—breakfast is the most important meal of the day! Everyone who wants to maintain a healthy lifestyle should eat breakfast consistently to power them through the day. Of course, not everyone has a ton of time in the morning to fix an elaborate meal, so I've included several quick and easy breakfast recipes for even the most time-crunched people. Eat up!

Oatmeal Three Ways

Oatmeal is so versatile—here are three of my favorites!

Maple-Meal
½ cup oatmeal, dry
¼ cup sugar-free maple syrup
5 sprays I Can't Believe It's Not Butter! spray
¼ cup nonfat milk
Dash cinnamon
1 packet Splenda

Cook oatmeal according to directions. Add syrup and I Can't Believe It's Not Butter! spray, and mix well. Top with milk, cinnamon, and Splenda to taste.

Makes: 1 serving

Per serving: calories 194; fat 3 grams; carbs 35 grams; protein 8 grams; fiber 4 grams

Fresh 'n' Fruity
    ½ cup oatmeal, dry
    1 tablespoon sugar-free apricot or blackberry jam
    1 packet Splenda
    ¼ cup nonfat milk

Cook oatmeal according to directions. Add jam, Splenda, and milk. Mix and serve.

Makes: 1 serving

Per serving: calories 190; fat 3 grams; carbs 36 grams; protein 8 grams; fiber 4 grams

Peanut Butter Bliss
    ½ cup oatmeal
    1 tablespoon reduced-fat chunky peanut butter
    2 tablespoons (or ½ minibox) raisins

Cook oatmeal according to directions. Mix in peanut butter and raisins and enjoy.

Makes: 1 serving

Per serving: calories 266; fat 9 grams; carbs 40 grams; protein 9 grams; fiber 5 grams

Magic Muffins
The perfect breakfast on the go!

Preheat oven to 375 degrees.

Combine these ingredients in a bowl:
    1½ cups oat bran
    1 cup natural bran cereal
    1 cup ground flaxseed meal
    1 cup vanilla protein powder
    1 tablespoon baking powder
    1 teaspoon baking soda
    ¼ teaspoon salt

Mix these ingredients in the blender:
    1 large or 2 small oranges cut into large pieces (skin and all!)
    1 cup Splenda granular
    ¼ cup sugar-free maple syrup
    1 cup reduced-fat buttermilk
    ½ cup no-sugar-added applesauce
    4 egg whites
    2 teaspoons cinnamon

Combine dry ingredients with blended ingredients and let sit for 10 minutes. Scoop into muffin tins and bake for 18–20 minutes.

Makes: 24 muffins

Serving size: 2 muffins

Per muffin: calories 159; fat 5 grams; protein 11 grams; carbs 23 grams; fiber 6 grams

Berri-licious Crepes
A Saturday morning treat!
    3 egg whites
    1 tablespoon skim milk
    2 tablespoons blueberry muffin mix, any brand
    ½ cup fat-free cottage cheese
    1 tablespoon berry fruit spread

Spray a large skillet or crepe pan with nonfat cooking spray and place over medium heat. Combine egg whites, milk, and muffin mix in a bowl, whisking until fluffy. Pour batter into pan in a thin layer. Cook for 1 minute, then flip over and cook for another minute. In a separate bowl, combine cottage cheese and fruit spread and microwave for 20–30 seconds. Flip cooked crepe onto a plate and pour cheese mixture into the center. Fold the ends of the crepe inward, roll it up, and enjoy.

Makes: 1 serving

Per serving: calories 310; fat 3 grams; protein 28 grams; carbs 40 grams; fiber 3 grams

BRIGHT IDEA
For an even sweeter treat, top with diced strawberries, blueberries, or other fresh fruit!

Strawberries and Cream

Super refreshing

    10 strawberries, diced

    4 ounces (1 container)
        Dannon Light & Fit Carb &
        Sugar Control vanilla cream
        yogurt

Layer strawberries and yogurt
in a bowl.

Makes: 1 serving

*Per serving: calories 82;
fat 3 grams; carbs 8 grams;
protein 6 grams; fiber 1 gram*

BRIGHT IDEA
Add a few tablespoons of your
favorite cereal for an extra crunch!

Yogurt Parfait

Quick and yummy

    ½ cup Kashi Go Lean
        Crunch! cereal

    ¾ cup blueberries

    4 ounces Dannon Light & Fit
        Carb & Sugar Control vanilla
        cream yogurt

Layer the ingredients in a bowl or
glass. Eat up!

Makes: 1 serving

*Per serving: Cal 194; fat 5 grams;
carbs 31 grams; protein 10 grams;
fiber 6 grams*

Early-Start Power Pita

For those hungry mornings

    4 large egg whites

    1 Morningstar brand breakfast
        patty

    1 slice fat-free cheese, cheddar
        or mozzarella

    ¼ cup salsa

    1 whole-wheat pita

Spray a skillet with nonstick cooking
spray and cook egg whites over
medium heat. Heat the breakfast
patty in the microwave as directed on
the package. Break up the patty with
a fork and knife and add to pan with
nearly cooked eggs. Add the cheese
and salsa and cook until cheese
is melted. Stuff into a toasted pita.

Makes: 1 serving

*Per serving: calories 375;
fat 5 grams; carbs 43 grams;
protein 37 grams; fiber 7 grams*

Breakfast Pizza

Add a little *abondanza* to your
morning!

    1 whole-wheat tortilla

    4 egg whites

    ¼ cup marinara sauce

    2 tablespoons shredded
        Parmesan cheese

Coat both sides of the tortilla and a
large skillet with nonfat cooking
spray. Heat the tortilla in the skillet,
turning frequently, until both
sides are crisp. Remove the tortilla
and set aside. Spray skillet once
more with nonstick spray and add

the egg whites. Cook eggs as a whole
(without scrambling) for 2–3 minutes on each side, or until golden
brown. Spread the marinara sauce
on the tortilla, then slide the eggs on
top. Cover with cheese and
microwave for 20–30 seconds or
until cheese is melted.

Makes: 1 serving

*Per pizza: calories 204; fat 9 grams;
carbs 29 grams; protein 18 grams;
fiber 15 grams*

Cozy Morning Grapefruit

A twist on an old favorite!

    1 pink grapefruit

    ½ teaspoon cinnamon

    1 teaspoon Splenda

    1 tablespoon sugar-free
        maple syrup

Cut grapefruit in half and bake in a
stove or toaster oven at 400 degrees
for 5 minutes. Remove and top with
cinnamon, Splenda, and syrup.

Makes: 1 serving

*Per serving: calories 88;
fat 0 grams; carbs 23 grams;
protein 2 grams; fiber 4 grams*

Blueberry Pancakes

A Biggest Loser favorite

- ½ cup oatmeal
- ½ cup reduced-fat buttermilk
- 1 egg white, lightly beaten
- ½ teaspoon baking soda
- ¼ teaspoon vanilla extract
- ¼ teaspoon salt
- ½ cup fresh blueberries
- I Can't Believe It's Not Butter! spray
- Sugar-free pancake syrup

Pour oatmeal in a blender and grind on high for 2 minutes or until oatmeal is finely chopped. Pour ground oatmeal into a large bowl and add buttermilk, egg white, baking soda, vanilla, and salt. Mix by hand until just blended. Gently stir in berries and let sit for 10 minutes. Heat a large skillet over medium heat and spray with nonfat cooking spray. Pour batter into skillet in ⅛-cup dollops. Cook for 2 minutes each side, or until pancakes are golden brown. Top with a few tablespoons of sugar-free syrup and a few squirts of I Can't Believe It's Not Butter! spray.

Makes: 1 serving (3–4 pancakes)

Per serving: calories 140; fat 3 grams; carbs 20 grams; protein 8 grams; fiber 3 grams

Kim's Breakfast Bar

Because they don't need to be refrigerated, these bars are great for traveling!

- 3½ cups rolled oats
- 1½ cups powdered nonfat milk
- 1 tablespoon cinnamon
- 1 cup sugar-free maple syrup
- 2 egg whites
- ¼ cup light orange juice
- 1 teaspoon vanilla

Preheat oven to 325 degrees. Combine oats, milk powder, and cinnamon in a bowl and mix well. In a separate bowl, whisk together syrup, egg whites, orange juice, and vanilla. Add to dry ingredients and mix well. Spray a cookie sheet with nonstick cooking spray. Spread oatmeal mixture in the pan to about ¼-inch thickness all around. Before cooking, cut the mixture into 10 separate bars with a sharp knife. Bake until golden brown, about 20–30 minutes. Remove and let cool thoroughly. Store bars in an airtight container.

Makes: 10 bars

Per bar: calories 250; fat 2 grams; carbs 35 grams; protein 10 grams; fiber 7 grams

LUNCH

When you think of lunch, you probably envision a boring old salad or a dry, flavorless sandwich. But lunch does not have to be humdrum! The more exciting you can make your lunch, the more likely you will be to eat it and keep your nutritional goals on track. Try some of these exciting options and make lunch fun again!

Tuna Salad with a Twist

A healthy twist on an old favorite

- 8 ounces (1 can) white tuna in water (preferably low sodium)
- 2 tablespoons low-fat mayo
- ¾ teaspoon lemon zest
- 1 squeeze of lemon juice
- 2 tablespoons chopped celery
- 2 tablespoons chopped green onion
- 1½ teaspoons celery seeds

Drain tuna and place in a large bowl. Add the rest of the ingredients and blend well. Chill for 1 hour and serve.

Makes: 2 servings

Per serving: calories 170; fat 3 grams; carbs 4 grams; protein 30 grams; fiber 2 grams

BRIGHT IDEA

This recipe is very versatile! Serve a scoop of tuna salad on a bed of greens, spread it on whole-wheat bread as a sandwich, or roll it in a whole-grain tortilla as a wrap!

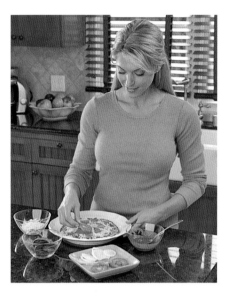

Personal Pizza

Fugghetaboutit! This pizza rocks!

- 1 low-carb flour tortilla
- ¼ cup low-fat marinara sauce
- ¼ cup reduced-fat mozzarella cheese
- 3 slices tomato
- ¼ cup fresh vegetable toppings of your choice (onion, mushrooms, bell peppers, etc.)
- 2 ounces thinly sliced cooked chicken breast

Coat a large skillet and both sides of the tortilla with nonfat cooking spray and cook until crispy. Remove tortilla from skillet and layer with marinara sauce, cheese, tomato, veggies, and chicken. Place in microwave or bake in toaster oven until veggies are soft and cheese is melted.

Makes: 1 serving

Per serving: calories 250; fat 8 grams; carbs 29 grams; protein 23 grams; fiber 14 grams

Curried Chicken Salad

Great as leftovers!

- 6-ounce can unsweetened pineapple juice
- 1 pound boneless, skinless chicken breasts
- ½ cup boiling water
- 4 tablespoons raisins or dried cranberries
- 1 medium onion, chopped
- 1 medium carrot, grated
- 1 tablespoon curry powder
- ½ teaspoon salt
- ¼ teaspoon ginger
- 5 tablespoons nonfat sugar-free vanilla yogurt

In a microwave-safe dish, pour pineapple juice over chicken. Cover and cook in microwave on high for 1 minute. Remove, turn chicken over, and microwave for another minute. Continue this process until chicken is no longer pink inside. Remove and let stand for 5 minutes. Pour water into a small pot and bring to a boil. Put raisins into a small bowl, and cover with boiling water. Set aside. Remove chicken from microwave dish, saving 2 tablespoons of the remaining pineapple juice, and cut chicken into bite-size pieces. Combine chicken, onion, carrot, curry powder, salt, ginger, reserved juice, and yogurt in a large bowl and mix well. Drain raisins and add to mixture, stirring thoroughly. Chill 2 hours. Serve over romaine lettuce.

Makes: 4 servings

Per serving: calories 179; fat 4 grams; protein 21 grams; carbs 20 grams; fiber 5 grams

Chicken Pita

A sandwich in a snap

- 1 chicken breast (6 ounces)
- 1 whole-wheat pita
- 1½ ounces low-fat feta cheese, crumbled
- ¼ cup chopped tomato
- 2 tablespoons chopped onion
- ¼ cup chopped cucumber
- Squeeze of lemon

Grill or bake the chicken and cut into bite-size pieces. Carefully open the pita and stuff with chicken, cheese, tomato, onion, and cucumber. Top with a squeeze of lemon.

Makes: 1 serving

Per serving: calories 490; fat 9 grams; protein 52 grams; carbs 41 grams; fiber 7 grams

BRIGHT IDEA

Make your own "hot pocket"! Heat the whole pita in the microwave oven for 30–45 seconds!

Chef Salad*

So good, you'll never miss the "real thing"!

- 4 ounces fat-free turkey breast, chopped
- 4 ounces extra-lean low-sodium ham, chopped
- 3 ounces fat-free mozzarella cheese, chopped
- ½ Roma tomato, chopped
- ¼ cup chopped hearts of palm
- ¼ avocado, diced
- 2 cups chopped romaine lettuce
- 3 tablespoons low-fat ranch dressing

In a large bowl, toss meats, cheese, and vegetables together. Add lettuce and toss again. Drizzle with dressing and serve.

Makes: 2 servings

Per serving: calories 234; fat 4.5 grams; protein 37 grams; carbs 11 grams; fiber 5 grams

Turkey Wrap*

My all-too-frequent in-the-car lunch

- 1 tablespoon light mayo
- 1 teaspoon mustard
- 1 low-carb whole-wheat tortilla
- 8 ounces lean sliced turkey breast
- 1 cup sliced veggies of your choice (bell peppers, cucumber, sprouts, pickles, etc.)

Spread mayo and mustard on the tortilla. Add turkey and veggies in the center, and roll it up.

Makes: 1 serving

Per serving: calories 263; fat 12 grams; carbs 16 grams; protein 27 grams; fiber 7 grams

---

BRIGHT IDEA

For a wrap with an exotic twist, trade the mayo and mustard for a dollop of plain yogurt or a tablespoon of hummus and a few sprigs of fresh herbs such as cilantro, basil, or thyme!

The Best-Ever Burrito*

Taco Bell's got nothing on these!

- 4 ounces extra-lean ground turkey
- 1 tablespoon chili powder
- ½ cup fat-free refried beans
- 1 large onion slice, chopped
- 2 whole-grain low-carb tortillas
- 1 slice fat-free cheddar or pepper jack cheese
- 2 tablespoons canned chopped green chilies
- 2 tablespoons salsa

Spray a large skillet with nonfat cooking spray and place over medium heat. Add turkey and chili powder and cook until browned. Add refried beans and onion and heat in skillet until warm. Spread turkey mixture in tortillas and top with cheese, chilies, and salsa.

Makes: 2 servings

Per serving: calories 242; fat 4 grams; carbs 36 grams; protein 27 grams; fiber 17 grams

---

BRIGHT IDEA

Hey, you Taco Bell fans! Add a few packets of Taco Bell hot sauce to your burrito for a healthy fast-food fix!

Chicken Tortilla Soup

Satisfying and savory

- 28 ounces (2 cans) nonfat, reduced-sodium chicken broth
- 4 ounces (1 can) stewed tomatoes with juice
- 3 tablespoons chopped fresh cilantro
- 2 cups stir-fry veggies (peppers, onions, mushrooms, bok choy, sprouts)
- 2 cups chopped cooked chicken
- 1 cup baked tortilla chips, crushed

In a large saucepan, combine chicken broth, stewed tomatoes, cilantro, and vegetables, and bring to a boil. Reduce heat, cover, and simmer for 3 minutes. Add chicken and cook for 2 minutes or until chicken is heated through. Spoon into 4 bowls and top each with ¼ cup of crushed chips.

Makes: 4 servings

Per serving: calories 247; fat 6 grams; carbs 17 grams; protein 24 grams; fiber 2 grams

BRIGHT IDEA

For additional Mexican flair, top soup with a tablespoon of light sour cream, a dash of hot sauce, or ¼ cup chopped avocado!

Mom's Chicken Bits

Yes, even my mommy has gone healthy!

- 1 teaspoon paprika
- ⅔ cup crushed reduced-fat Ritz crackers
- ½ teaspoon garlic powder
- ½ teaspoon dried oregano
- ⅛ teaspoon pepper
- 1 pound boneless, skinless chicken breasts, diced
- 1 egg white, lightly beaten

Preheat oven to 450 degrees. Put paprika, crushed Ritz crackers, garlic powder, oregano, and pepper into a large Ziploc bag and shake well. Place chicken pieces in a bowl with the egg white and mix well so the chicken is thoroughly coated. Put a few pieces of chicken at a time into the Ziploc bag and shake to coat evenly. Place coated pieces in a single layer on a cookie sheet sprayed with nonstick cooking spray and bake 7–9 minutes or until chicken is no longer pink.

Makes: 4 servings

Per serving: calories 191; fat 2 grams; protein 29 grams; carbs 13 grams; fiber 0 grams

The Fast-Food-Cure Cheeseburger—with Secret Sauce!

Look out, Micky-Dee's— this burger's got it going on!

Burger:

- 4 ounces extra-lean ground beef or turkey
- 1 whole-wheat hamburger bun
- 1 fat-free cheddar cheese slice

Secret Sauce:

- 1 teaspoon dill relish
- 1 teaspoon reduced-fat mayo
- 1 teaspoon honey mustard
- ¼ teaspoon Worcestershire sauce

Shape ground beef or turkey into a large patty. Grill or cook the patty in a pan with nonfat cooking spray until done. Reduce grill or stove heat and place cheese slice on top of patty to melt. Combine secret sauce ingredients and spread on either side of a toasted bun. Put burger into bun and enjoy!

Makes: 1 serving

Per serving: calories 390; fat 7 grams; protein 34 grams; carbs 42 grams; fiber 4 grams

BRIGHT IDEA

For a deluxe burger, add the usual burger fixin's: a slice of tomato, a round of onion, and a big leaf of lettuce or even a handful of baby spinach leaves!

Three-Bean Super Salad*

Great as a meal or as a side dish

- ⅓ cup Splenda
- 2 tablespoons olive oil
- ½ cup white wine vinegar
- 1 can (15 ounces) lima beans, rinsed and drained
- 1 can (15 ounces) red kidney beans, rinsed and drained
- 1 can (15 ounces) garbanzo beans, rinsed and drained
- 4 cloves garlic, minced
- ½ cup sliced hearts of palm
- ½ cup artichoke hearts (in water)
- ½ cup minced red onion
- ¾ cup chopped fresh parsley
- ¼ cup chopped fresh cilantro

Whisk the Splenda, olive oil, and vinegar together in a bowl. Add remaining ingredients and mix well. Refrigerate overnight.

Makes: 10 servings

Per serving: calories 160; fat 4 grams; protein 7 grams; carbs 25 grams; fiber 7 grams

SIDE DISHES

Many times, you'll barbecue a big batch of chicken or roast a pork loin and will be in need of a side to accompany it. Instead of always steaming your veggies or eating them raw, try some of these terrific side dishes for a change of pace. They're guaranteed to please even the most veggie-adverse palate (e.g., your super-choosy ten-year-old)!

Veggie Ceviche

A favorite appetizer at parties

- 1 can (14 ounces) artichoke hearts in water, drained and chopped
- 1 large tomato, seeded and chopped
- ¼ pound white mushrooms, chopped
- ⅓ cup chopped scallions
- ¼ cup fresh lime juice
- ⅛ cup vegetable oil
- Salt, cayenne pepper, and black pepper to taste
- 1 ripe avocado, peeled, pitted, chopped

Combine all ingredients except avocado in a large bowl and mix well. Marinate for 1 hour. Add chopped avocado, mix, and serve.

Makes: 8 servings

Per serving: calories 87; fat 7 grams; protein 2 grams; carbs 5 grams; fiber 3 grams

---

BRIGHT IDEA

Serve ceviche with baked whole-wheat pita triangles! Cut a pita into wedges, spritz with I Can't Believe It's Not Butter! spray, and sprinkle with garlic powder. Bake in the oven at 400 degrees, turning frequently, until crispy.

Vegetable Gratin Casserole

Colorful and flavorful

- 2 cloves garlic, crushed
- 2 shallots, finely chopped
- 1 tablespoon chopped fresh basil
- ¼ teaspoon ground black pepper
- 2 yellow squash, sliced lengthwise
- 2 zucchinis, sliced lengthwise
- 3 tomatoes, seeded and sliced in rounds
- ½ teaspoon salt
- 2 tablespoons low-fat or fat-free grated Parmesan cheese
- ¼ cup low-fat dry breadcrumbs

Preheat oven to 400 degrees. Spray an 8-inch-square baking dish with nonfat cooking spray. Combine the garlic, shallots, basil, and pepper, and spread this mixture in the bottom of the dish. Layer the yellow squash, zucchini, and tomatoes in the dish, sprinkling each layer with a little salt. Sprinkle the top with cheese and bread crumbs. Bake for 40–45 minutes, or until vegetables are tender.

Makes: 4 servings

Per serving: calories 107; fat 1 gram; protein 3.5 grams; carbs 24 grams; fiber 4 grams

Oven-"Fried" Sweet Potatoes
Great taste without the grease
- 3 medium sweet potatoes
- 1 tablespoon olive oil
- 1 teaspoon oregano
- ½ teaspoon black pepper

Scrub potatoes and cut into lengthwise wedges. Place strips in a bowl of cold water and let stand for 30 minutes. Drain and pat dry. Preheat oven to 400 degrees. Place potatoes and oil in a bowl and toss to coat evenly. Spread potatoes on a baking sheet and sprinkle with oregano and black pepper. Bake for 45 minutes, turning potatoes halfway through to brown on both sides.

Makes: 3 servings

Per serving: calories 95; fat 4 grams; protein 1 gram; carbs 13 grams; fiber 2 grams

BRIGHT IDEA
Sprinkle cooked sweet potatoes with malt vinegar for that fish 'n' chips flavor!

Baby Lemon Green Beans
Refreshing and crisp
- 1 pound fresh baby green beans
- ½ cup chopped red bell pepper
- 2 tablespoons lemon juice
- ½ teaspoon dried basil
- 2 teaspoons toasted sesame seeds

Put green beans, red pepper, and basil in a vegetable steamer. Steam for 3–5 minutes, or until vegetables are crisp-tender. Toss veggies with lemon juice, basil, and sesame seeds. Serve hot or chilled.

Makes: 4 servings

Per serving: calories 31; fat 0.5 gram; protein 2 grams; carbs 7 grams; fiber 3 grams

Cauliflower Casserole
This dish will make you fall in love with cauliflower!
- 1 cup chopped mushrooms
- 3 cups chopped cauliflower
- ½ cup chopped sweet onions
- 1 tablespoon olive oil
- 2 teaspoons apple cider vinegar
- 2 teaspoons lemon juice
- ¼ teaspoon ground pepper
- ½ teaspoon salt
- 2 cloves garlic, crushed
- ¼ cup finely chopped chives

Preheat oven to 350 degrees. Spray a baking dish with nonfat cooking spray. Combine all ingredients and spread evenly in the baking dish. Bake uncovered for 45 minutes, stirring a few times to prevent burning.

Makes: 4 servings

Per serving: calories 64; fat 4 grams; protein 2.5 grams; carbs 7 grams; fiber 2.5 grams

Sesame Sugar Snap Peas
A sure-fire family favorite
- 1 pound sugar snap peas
- 1 teaspoon toasted sesame seeds
- 1 teaspoon sesame oil

Steam peas for 3–5 minutes. Toss in a large bowl with sesame seeds and oil and serve hot.

Makes: 4 servings

Per serving: calories 42; fat 1 gram; protein 2 grams; carbs 6 grams; fiber 2 grams

BRIGHT IDEA
These peas are also a great addition to a salad! Chill a few and add them to your lunchtime salad for an oriental crunch.

Roasted Asparagus
A great alternative to steaming
- 1 pound fresh asparagus, trimmed
- 1 teaspoon olive oil
- 1 tablespoon balsamic vinegar

Preheat oven to 500 degrees. In a shallow baking pan, toss asparagus with oil until coated. Roast asparagus in oven until tender (about 10 minutes), shaking pan every few minutes. Remove and drizzle with balsamic vinegar.

Makes: 6 servings

Per serving: calories 22; fat 1 gram; protein 2 grams; carbs 3 grams; fiber 1.5 grams

Hot German Potato Salad

So good, everyone will want your "secret" potato salad recipe!

- 1½ pounds new red skinned potatoes
- 3 tablespoons Splenda
- 1 teaspoon white flour
- ¼ teaspoon salt
- 1 tablespoon canola oil
- 4 thin deli slices of lean ham, cut into small pieces
- ½ cup chopped onion
- ½ cup water
- ⅓ cup white vinegar
- 2 tablespoons chopped fresh parsley

Fill a large pot with water. Wash and quarter potatoes and add to pot. Bring water and potatoes to a boil and cook until potatoes are easily pierced with a fork (20–25 minutes). Drain and set aside in a large bowl. Combine Splenda, flour, and salt in a small bowl and set aside. Place oil in a large skillet over medium heat. Add ham and cook until lightly browned. Add onion and sauté with ham until translucent. Add Splenda mixture to skillet, and cook for about 1 minute. Add water and vinegar, stirring constantly for 2–3 minutes or until nearly boiling. Pour skillet mixture over hot potatoes. Add chopped parsley, mix thoroughly, and serve.

Makes: 8 servings

Per serving: calories 110; fat 4 grams; carbs 17 grams; protein 3 grams; fiber 2 grams

Spanish Rice*

Healthy brown rice with a kick!

- 1½ cups chicken stock
- 3 tablespoons olive oil
- 1 large onion, chopped
- 1 cup chopped green bell pepper
- 1 clove garlic, crushed
- 1½ cups brown rice
- 1 can (28 ounces) crushed tomatoes with liquid
- ½ cup chopped mushrooms

Place chicken stock in a small saucepot and bring to a boil. In a large saucepot, heat oil and cook onion and bell pepper until tender. Add garlic, sautéing for a few minutes. Add the raw rice and cook for 5 minutes, stirring frequently. Add tomatoes and boiling chicken stock to rice mixture and bring to a boil. Cover and reduce heat. Add mushrooms and simmer until the rice has absorbed the liquid and is tender.

Note: Depending on the kind of rice you use, you may have to add more water or stock as the rice cooks to make it soft and tender.

Makes: 8 servings (½ cup)

Per serving: calories 293; fat 9 grams; saturated fat 1 gram; protein 7 grams; carbs 50; fiber 5 grams

DINNER

I don't know about you, but dinner was a big deal in my family. Every night we'd sit down at the dinner table to a home-cooked meal and would spend some quality family time together. I have come up with several healthy dinner options that are reminiscent of those days. Even the most finicky families can enjoy them together! Now when your family asks, *Hey what's for dinner?* you'll get cheers instead of sneers!

Turkey Meatloaf

Your mother's meatloaf was never this good!

- 1 teaspoon instant chicken bouillon
- ½ cup salsa
- 1½ pounds extra-lean ground turkey
- ¾ cup quick oatmeal
- ½ cup chopped onion
- 2 teaspoons dried basil
- ½ teaspoon garlic powder
- ¼ teaspoon black pepper
- 1 egg white

Preheat oven to 350 degrees. Combine all ingredients in a large bowl, mixing well. Pack mixture into an 8-inch by 4-inch loaf pan. Cook for 1 hour, or until the center of the loaf is no longer pink.

Makes: 6 servings

Per serving: calories 173; fat 2 grams; protein 28 grams; carbs 9 grams; fiber 2 grams

Lasagna*

The healthiest lasagna you'll ever love!

1 pound lean ground turkey
1 cup chopped onion
3 lean Italian sausage links, chopped
2 cloves garlic, crushed
2 cups sliced mushrooms
4 tablespoons Italian seasoning
1 large container (1 pound, 8 ounces) fat-free cottage cheese
1 jar (26 ounces) low-fat marinara sauce
6 lasagna noodles, boiled and cooled
1 bag spinach leaves, chopped
1 container (15 ounces) fat-free ricotta cheese
1 cup fat-free Parmesan cheese

Preheat oven to 375 degrees. In a large pan, cook turkey, onions, sausage, garlic, and mushrooms until turkey is browned and veggies are soft. Set aside. In a small bowl, combine Italian seasoning and cottage cheese and set aside. Spray a lasagna pan with nonfat cooking spray. Layer with lasagna ingredients in this order: ⅓ jar marinara sauce, 2 noodles, ½ bag of chopped spinach, ½ container ricotta cheese, ⅓ jar marinara sauce, ½ cottage cheese mixture, 2 noodles, meat mixture, ½ bag of chopped spinach, remaining ricotta cheese, ⅓ jar marinara sauce, remaining cottage cheese mixture, 2 noodles, Parmesan cheese. Bake 50–60 minutes. Let stand 15 minutes before serving.

Makes: 12 Servings

Per serving: calories 300; fat 6 grams; protein 28 grams; carbs 33 grams; fiber 3 grams

---

BRIGHT IDEA

Pack yourself, your spouse, or your kids a little leftover lasagna love for lunch! Put a wedge of lasagna in a small Tupperware and nuke it at lunchtime.

Flank Steak with Brown Sugar Rub

A beef-lover's dream!

1 tablespoon Splenda Brown Sugar Blend
1 teaspoon salt
¾ teaspoon ground cumin
3 cloves garlic, crushed
1½ pounds flank steak, trimmed and rinsed

Preheat a grill to medium high. Combine Splenda Brown Sugar Blend, salt, cumin, and garlic into a paste. Rub steak with mixture and let sit for 15 minutes. Grill steak 5–10 minutes each side, or until it reaches the desired degree of doneness.

Makes: 7 servings

Per serving: calories 165; fat 7 grams; protein 21 grams; carbs 2 grams; 0 fiber

---

BRIGHT IDEA
These leftovers make great sandwiches!

Grilled Halibut Amandine

Fresh herbs make this dish unbeatable!

¼ cup fresh parsley
2 tablespoons chopped fresh thyme
1 tablespoon black pepper
3 cloves garlic, crushed
1 teaspoon freshly grated lemon peel
3 tablespoons lemon juice
¼ cup sliced almonds, toasted
4–6 ounces halibut filets

Preheat grill to medium-low heat. Combine parsley, thyme, pepper, garlic, lemon peel, and lemon juice and puree in a food processor. Spread mixture over each filet and let marinate for 10 minutes. Place filets on grill and cook 4–6 minutes on each side, or until fish flakes easily with a fork. Sprinkle cooked fish with almonds.

Makes: 4 servings

Per serving: calories 274; fat 11 grams; protein 38 grams; carbs 4 grams; fiber 2 grams

Grilled Lemon Chicken and Veggie Salad

Light, lemony, and fabulous

Marinade

¾ cup fresh lemon juice
¼ cup olive oil
1 tablespoon fresh chopped thyme leaves
1 teaspoon salt

Salad

4 chicken breasts (6 ounces each)
1 cup sugar snap peas, cooked
½ red pepper, cut into strips
½ yellow pepper, cut into strips
½ cup chopped and seeded tomatoes
½ zucchini, cut into strips
2 tablespoons fresh chopped cilantro
1 tablespoon olive oil
¼ teaspoon salt
¼ teaspoon black pepper
1 head romaine lettuce, washed and chopped
Squeeze of fresh lemon juice

Combine chicken marinade ingredients in a large Ziploc bag. Place chicken in bag, seal, and marinate in the refrigerator for an hour. Occasionally shake the bag to distribute the marinade evenly. Grill marinated chicken on a medium-high grill. Cut into strips and cool. Combine peas, red and yellow peppers, tomatoes, and zucchini with cilantro, olive oil, salt, and pepper. Mix chicken strips with veggies and serve on a bed of romaine lettuce. Top with a squeeze of fresh lemon juice.

Makes: 4 servings

Per serving: calories 261; fat 7 grams; protein 41 grams; carbs 8 grams; fiber 2 grams

Shrimp Diablo

Sinfully spicy!

1 tablespoon olive oil
¼ cup lemon juice
1 tablespoon Cajun seasoning (preferably salt free)
1 clove garlic, crushed
1 pound medium raw shrimp, deveined, tail on

Soak 6–8 wooden skewers in cold water for 30 minutes. Combine olive oil, lemon juice, Cajun seasoning, and garlic in a small bowl. Rinse and shell shrimp, leaving the tails on. Place shrimp in a large plastic baggie or Tupperware and pour in marinade, shaking to distribute evenly. Marinate for 15–30 minutes. Preheat grill to medium. Thread shrimp on skewers. Grill for 2–3 minutes on each side.

Makes: 4 servings

Per serving: calories 170; fat 6 grams; protein 26 grams; carbs 3 grams; fiber 0 grams

BRIGHT IDEA

These shrimp are great on a salad, over rice, or as an appetizer!

Chicken Cacciatore

A healthy twist on traditional cuisine

2 tablespoons olive oil
1 clove garlic, crushed
6 boneless, skinless chicken breasts
1 medium onion, chopped
2 tablespoons chopped green pepper
4 tomatoes, seeded and chopped
¼ cup dry white wine
¼ teaspoon rosemary
1 bay leaf
¼ teaspoon basil
⅛ teaspoon black pepper

Heat oil and sauté garlic in a large skillet over medium heat. Add chicken and brown both sides. Remove chicken and put onion and green pepper into pan, sautéing until tender. Return chicken to skillet and add remaining ingredients. Simmer over low heat for 30 minutes. Remove bay leaf and serve.

Makes: 6 servings

Per serving: calories 267; fat 6 grams; protein 46 grams; carbs 29 grams; fiber 1 gram

Asian Salmon*

The unique marinade makes this dish moist and flavorful.

- ¼ cup low-sodium soy sauce
- 2 tablespoons apricot-pineapple preserves
- 2 cloves garlic, crushed
- 2 teaspoons rice vinegar
- ½ teaspoon grated fresh ginger
- ¼ teaspoon red pepper flakes
- 4 salmon filets (6 ounces each), skinned

Preheat grill to medium heat. Whisk together marinade ingredients in a small bowl. Score each salmon filet diagonally on both sides with a sharp knife, about ¼-inch deep, so the marinade can soak in. Place fish on grill and spoon sauce onto each filet. Cook for 4–5 minutes, then turn over, add more marinade to each filet, and grill for 4–5 more minutes, or until fish flakes easily with a fork.

Makes: 4 servings (6 ounces each)

Per serving: calories 390; fat 21 grams; protein 39 grams; carbs 8 grams; fiber 0 grams

Ginger Chicken and Broccoli

Better than Chinese takeout!

- 1 tablespoon olive oil
- ⅛ teaspoon garlic, crushed
- 1 teaspoon fresh ginger, grated
- 4 boneless skinless chicken breasts, cut into strips
- ⅛ teaspoon black pepper
- 6 cups broccoli florets
- 4½ cups snow peas
- 1¼ yellow onions, chopped
- 1½ tablespoons low sodium soy sauce
- ½ cup water

Heat olive oil in a wok or large non-stick skillet on medium heat. Add garlic and ginger and sauté for 1 minute. Add chicken and black pepper and sauté, tossing frequently, until meat is lightly browned (3–5 minutes). Add vegetables, soy sauce, and water, and continue cooking, stirring often, until the chicken is cooked through, the water is reduced, and the vegetables are tender (20 minutes).

Makes: 4 servings

Per serving: calories 251; fat 5 grams; protein 39 grams; carbs 14 grams; fiber 4 grams

Excellent Enchiladas*

My favorite Mexican recipe ever!

- 1 chicken bouillon cube
- 4 cups water
- 4 chicken breasts
- 1 can reduced-fat cream of chicken soup
- ½ cup fat-free sour cream
- 1 can green chilies
- ½ cup reduced-fat cheese, shredded, divided
- 1 can green chili enchilada sauce, divided
- 12 6-inch corn tortillas

Preheat oven to 350 degrees. Dissolve bouillon cube in 4 cups of boiling water. Add chicken and continue to boil for 20–30 minutes. Remove chicken and let cool. Combine 1 cup of remaining chicken bouillon water, chicken soup, sour cream, green chilies, ¼ cup of cheese, and all but ½ cup enchilada sauce in a large bowl. Shred chicken with a fork and add it to the bowl. Mix well. Roll chicken mixture into corn tortillas. Pour remaining enchilada sauce over rolled enchiladas and sprinkle with remaining cheese. Bake for 15 minutes or until cheese is melted.

Makes: 6 servings (2 enchiladas each)

Per serving: calories 315; fat 5 grams; protein 37 grams; carbs 29 grams; fiber 4 grams

DESSERT

Yes! You can fit dessert into your healthy lifestyle! Here are some creative ways I came up with for satisfying my sweet tooth without compromising my diet.

Grilled Fruit Kebob with Maple Glaze

Light in calories but heavy in flavor!

Fruit

- 2 large bananas, cut into rounds
- 6 kiwis, peeled and quartered lengthwise
- 4 large pears, chopped into bite-size pieces
- 1 can pineapple chunks

Glaze

- ½ cup sugar-free maple syrup
- 1 tablespoon cinnamon
- ½ tablespoon allspice
- 1 tablespoon vanilla extract
- 3 tablespoons I Can't Believe It's Not Butter! spread

Soak 6 wooden skewers in water for 30 minutes and preheat grill to medium high. Combine glaze ingredients and pour into a small saucepan, heating the mixture on medium. Spear the fruit onto the skewers and grill for 3–4 minutes, turning frequently. Remove from grill and drizzle glaze over cooked fruit.

Makes: 6 servings

Per serving: calories 30; fat 0 grams; carbs 4 grams; protein 0 grams; fiber 2 grams

Ginger Cookies

These are so good, you'll never know they're good for you!

- 2 cups whole-wheat flour (or 1 cup white and 1 cup whole wheat)
- 2 teaspoons baking soda
- 1 dash salt
- 2 teaspoons ground ginger
- 1 teaspoon ground cinnamon
- 1 cup Splenda Brown Sugar Blend
- 2 tablespoons light butter
- ¼ cup molasses
- 2 egg whites
- ½ cup unsweetened or no-sugar-added applesauce

Preheat the oven to 325 degrees. Combine the flour, baking soda, salt, ginger, cinnamon, and Splenda Brown Sugar Blend in a bowl and mix well by hand. In another large bowl, beat butter, molasses, egg whites, and applesauce on high using an electric mixer. Add dry ingredients and mix well by hand. Spray a baking sheet with nonfat cooking spray and drop the batter onto the sheet in teaspoons. (*Note*: These cookies spread *a lot*, so leave plenty of room in between! I recommend putting no more than nine cookies on a sheet at one time.) Bake 12–15 minutes or until cookies start to brown on the bottom. Cool on a rack or paper towels and serve right away.

Makes: 45 small–medium cookies

Serving size: 2 cookies

Per serving: calories 78; fat 1 gram; carbs 15 grams; protein 2 grams; fiber 2 grams

---

BRIGHT IDEA

For a healthy "ice cream sandwich," sandwich 2 tablespoons of Cool Whip Free topping between two Ginger Cookies, seal in a Ziploc baggie, and freeze overnight.

Banana Split Crunch

A Red Team favorite!

- 1 tablespoon sugar-free strawberry preserves
- 1 plain rice cake
- ½ small banana, sliced
- ¼ cup fat-free sugar-free instant chocolate pudding
- ½ cup fat-free no-sugar-added vanilla ice cream

Spread the preserves on the rice cake and top with sliced banana, chocolate pudding and ice cream.

Makes: 1 serving

Per serving: calories 211; fat 4 grams; protein 5 grams; carbs 47 grams; fiber 8 grams

Chewy Oatmeal Cookies

So good for you, you could eat them for breakfast!

- 2 cups quick oatmeal
- ½ cup all-natural, no-sugar-added applesauce
- 1 cup Splenda Brown Sugar Blend
- 2 egg whites
- ¼ teaspoon salt
- ½ teaspoon almond extract
- ½ cup finely chopped dates
- ½ cup finely chopped walnuts

Preheat oven to 350 degrees. Combine oatmeal, applesauce, and Splenda Brown Sugar Blend in a large bowl. In a separate bowl, beat egg whites until frothy, then add to the oatmeal mixture. Stir in salt, almond extract, dates, and walnuts. Drop by teaspoonfuls on baking sheets sprayed with nonfat cooking spray. Bake for 15 minutes or until the cookies begin to brown on the bottom. Cool on a rack.

Makes: 30 cookies

Serving size: 2 cookies

Per serving: calories 120; fat 3 grams; carbs 21 grams; protein 3 grams; fiber 2 grams

White Chiffon Cake

A great alternative to store-bought birthday cakes

- 2½ cups white cake flour
- 1½ cups Splenda granular
- 1 tablespoon baking powder
- 1 teaspoon salt
- 2 egg yolks
- ¾ cup water
- 1 teaspoon vanilla extract
- ½ cup no-sugar-added, all-natural applesauce
- 8 large egg whites
- 1 teaspoon cream of tartar

Preheat oven to 325 degrees. In a large bowl, combine flour, Splenda, baking powder, and salt. Add egg yolks, water, vanilla, and applesauce and beat with an electric mixer on high for 30 seconds or until smooth. Set aside. In a separate bowl, combine egg whites and cream of tartar. Beat on high until stiff peaks form (about 3 minutes). Gently fold the beaten egg whites into the batter. Pour batter into a 10-inch tube pan and bake for 60 minutes. Cool and serve solo, or topped with fat-free Cool Whip and a few strawberries.

Makes: 12 servings

Per serving: calories 150; fat 2 grams; carbs 19 grams; protein 4 grams; fiber 0 grams

Cherry Almond Cheesecake Tarts

These are my all-time favorite!

Crust
- 1½ cups white flour
- 1 cup quick oatmeal
- ¾ cup Splenda
- ¾ cup light margarine
- 1½ cups fat-free sour cream
- ½ teaspoon baking soda

Filling
- 8 ounces fat-free cream cheese
- ¼ cup Splenda
- ½ teaspoon almond extract
- 1 whole egg, lightly beaten
- ½ cup canned light cherry pie filling
- ½ cup sliced almonds

Preheat oven to 350 degrees. Combine flour, oatmeal, and Splenda in a bowl. Add margarine, sour cream, and baking soda and mix with a fork to make a thick paste. Spread 2 tablespoons each of this mixture evenly onto the bottoms and sides of 12 large muffin cups.

Mix the cream cheese, Splenda, and almond extract with an electric beater on medium until combined. Add the egg and mix again. Spoon this filling into the crust-lined muffin cups. Top each with a bit of cherry pie filling and a few almonds. Bake for 45–50 minutes. Cool before serving.

Makes: 12 tarts

Per tart: calories 150; fat 4 grams; carbs 20 grams; protein 5 grams; fiber 3 grams

Chocolate Chai Tea

Great for chilly winter evenings

  ½ cup boiling water
  1 black tea bag
  3 tablespoons Splenda
  2 tablespoons unsweetened
    Dutch cocoa powder
  2 cups nonfat lactose-free milk
  1 teaspoon vanilla extract
  ½ teaspoon ground cinnamon
  ½ teaspoon ground nutmeg
  Fat-free whipped cream
  Cinnamon stick

Bring the water to a boil in a small saucepan. Remove from heat, add the tea bag, cover, and steep for 3–5 minutes. Remove the bag and stir in Splenda and cocoa. Return to stove and bring the mixture to a boil over medium heat. Stir in milk, vanilla, cinnamon, and nutmeg. Cook until hot but not boiling. Pour the tea into a mug and garnish with some whipped cream and a cinnamon stick.

Makes: 2 servings

Per serving: calories 50; fat 0 grams; carbs 7.5 grams; protein 5 grams; fiber 0 grams

BRIGHT IDEA

To make recipes creamier, use lactose-free milk!

Apple "Almost" Pie

My husband's favorite treat

  1 teaspoon cinnamon
  ¼ cup sugar-free maple syrup
  ¼ cup water
  ½ teaspoon vanilla extract
  1 teaspoon Splenda Brown
    Sugar Blend
  1 large Granny Smith apple,
    sliced thin
  2 low-fat cinnamon graham
    cracker sheets, smashed,
    divided
  ½ cup fat-free, no-sugar-added
    vanilla ice cream

In a bowl, combine cinnamon, syrup, water, vanilla extract, and Splenda. Add apple slices and toss until evenly coated. Coat a skillet with nonfat cooking spray and cook apple mixture over medium heat until apples are tender and liquid is almost gone. Place ¼ of the smashed graham cracker in the bottom of two bowls and top with the apple mixture. Add ¼ cup of ice cream to each bowl and sprinkle the remaining graham crackers on top.

Makes: 2 servings

Per serving: calories 202; fat 2 grams; protein 3 grams; carbs 44 grams; fiber 4 grams

Peanut Butter Frozen Treat

This will cure anyone's sweet tooth!

  2 reduced-fat graham cracker
    sheets
  ½ tablespoon reduced-fat
    peanut butter
  2 tablespoons Cool Whip Free
    whipped topping

Spread the peanut butter on one graham cracker sheet and Cool Whip Free on the other sheet. Sandwich together and place in a Ziploc baggie. Freeze overnight.

Makes: 1 serving

Per serving: calories 188; fat 5 grams; protein 4 grams; carbs 32 grams; fiber 2 grams

Sweet Cinnamon Tortilla

Sounds weird, but it's surprisingly good!

  1 low-carb tortilla
  1 teaspoon cinnamon
  1 teaspoon Splenda
  I Can't Believe It's Not
    Butter! spray

Preheat skillet on medium. Spritz each side of the tortilla with 5 squirts of I Can't Believe It's Not Butter! spray. Cook in skillet, turning frequently, until crunchy and brown on both sides. Remove tortilla and squirt one side twice with I Can't Believe It's Not Butter! spray, then sprinkle with Splenda and cinnamon.

Makes: 1 serving

Per serving: calories 67; fat 3 grams; protein 5 grams; carbs 14 grams; fiber 10 grams

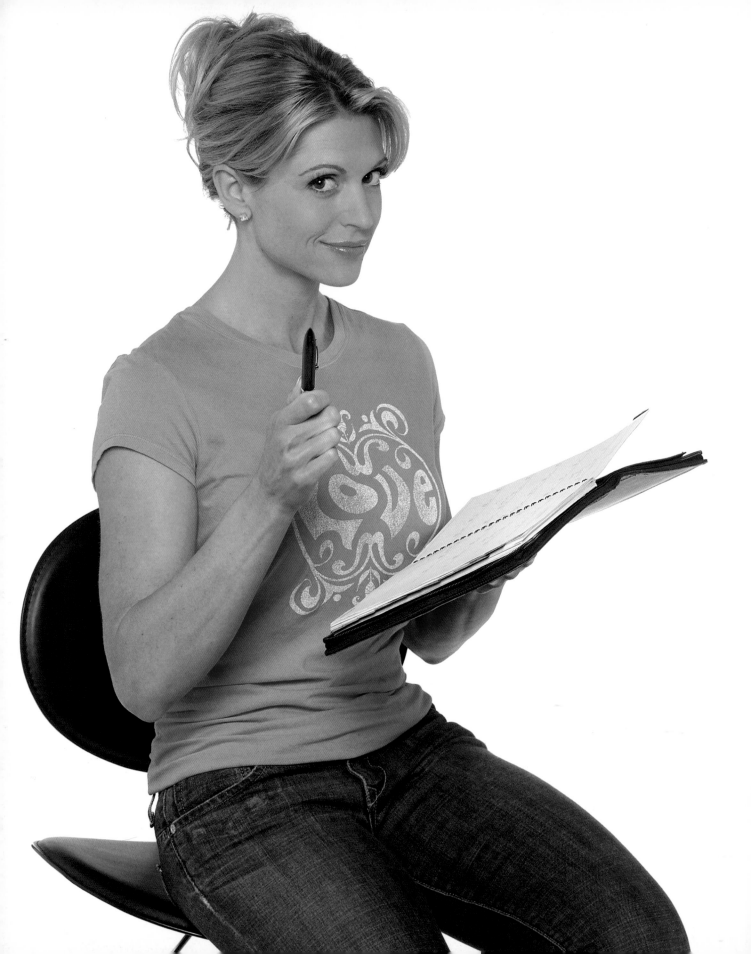

Your Future

CONGRATULATIONS! If you're reading this section, you've finished your twelve-week program and are feeling great! You should be really proud of yourself. It's so, *so* hard to make a commitment to change and follow through with it; you've done what so many people only talk about doing, and you've done it well! You've established a new lifestyle and have solidified some incredible healthy habits, and I bet you can't imagine your life without exercise and good nutrition!

Now you're probably wondering, what's next? What do I do now that I have reached my goal? This section is dedicated to helping you plan your future with fitness.

CHAPTER 17

Reassess and Reevaluate

Rewind

For more ideas on rewards, turn to Chapter 4, page 27.

Yippee! You've successfully completed your initial *Your Body, Your Life* twelve-week lifestyle transformation! I bet you look and feel completely differently than you did three months ago. You're probably smaller, leaner, and more energetic than ever before, and you're probably getting tons of comments and questions about your hot new bod! Hopefully you've also experienced an incredible mental evolution, shedding your negative self-image and changing your attitude toward yourself and your body. Whereas many people start this program full of self-doubt, most finish with a sense of purpose, accomplishment, and pride.

While mental progress is difficult to measure, physical progress is not. Remember back in Chapter 6 when you measured and weighed yourself and took those fitness tests? It's time to do that again, only this time I know you'll be pleased with the results!

RETEST AND REWARD

Open your journal to your Results page, or get out the piece of paper on which you recorded your original test results. Turn back to Chapter 6, carefully reread the directions for taking the fitness tests and measuring and weighing yourself, then retake each of those tests. Mark your new results underneath your original scores. See a difference? I bet you do!

Spend a little time thinking about what these new numbers mean to you. For some, they mean the beginning of a long journey toward substantial weight loss and a healthier lifestyle. For others they mean another step closer to beating diabetes. Whatever they mean to you, congratulate yourself heartily. It's not easy to accomplish what you've done, and you should be very proud of yourself!

When you're done patting yourself on the back, get to work thinking about your reward! Every job well done deserves a reward, and your prize for changing your lifestyle should be huge! Take yourself on a trip, spend a day at the spa, or buy yourself a new outfit to glam up your new body! Anything that makes you feel really good about yourself and your accomplishment is a terrific reward.

JOURNAL REVIEW

You can learn a lot by looking back on your journals. I have journals from the last ten years that I refer to constantly. If I am trying to reach a certain goal I have reached in the past, I have only to look in my journal to see how I trained, ate, and felt during the process. I learn from my mistakes and improve on my methods according to what I recorded in my journal.

Reread your journals to find out how things are going with your fitness program. Here are a few common patterns you might notice.

- **Are you always tired when you train?**
  Everyone has natural rhythms—they have higher energy sometimes and lower energy at other times. See whether switching your workout time changes your energy level. You might also need to eat a meal or a snack closer to your workout time so you have enough energy to train. Have something light but nutritious to give you energy without giving you an upset stomach.

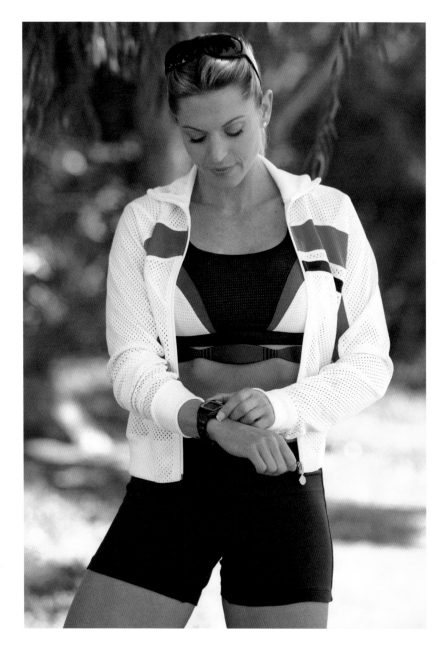

Rewind
For more information on Rest Days, turn to page 54!

- **Do you have insomnia?** If you work out in the evenings, that may be contributing to your problem, getting your body too fired up to be able to relax. Try training in the morning or early afternoon and see whether you notice a difference.
- **Are you always sore, stiff, and irritable?** You may be overtraining. Check your workout journal to see whether you're actively planning your Rest Days. If you're training five or more days in a row, you're overdoing it. Make a conscious effort to take at least two full days off from training every week if you're not already doing so.
- **Do you eat when you're sad, mad, or even glad?** Maybe you're an emotional eater, always putting something in your mouth when you're feeling highly emotional. Carefully reread your workout and food journals to see whether you can ID a pattern of emotional eating in your daily life.
- **Do you crave sugar a lot?** Perhaps you need to incorporate more dense foods into your diet such as vegetables, complex carbs, and protein that contain fiber and keep you fuller longer.
- **Do you always hit the vending machines in the afternoon?** Perhaps you need to eat more frequently during the day. Usually we go for chips, cookies, and other unhealthy snacks when we're depleted and our stomachs are empty. Keep your stomach full and your metabolism running by eating a meal or snack every 3–4 hours.

GOAL REVIEW

So you're done with your initial twelve weeks—now what? Your journey does not end here! In order to nurture your new healthy lifestyle, you've got to set some new goals. Most people are eager to make new goals after accomplishing their original ones, and feel like they can accomplish anything they set their minds to. I hope you feel this way, too!

Let's review the long-term goal examples I listed back in Chapter 4. Read each woman's story and see how their results helped dictate their next long-term goals.

Margie
Her Original Goal
"I will complete all twelve weeks of the *Your Body, Your Life* program, getting up an hour earlier to exercise before work four to five days a week. By this summer I will lose 10 pounds, will look great in a bikini, and will celebrate by taking a trip to Hawaii with my family!"

Her Story
Margie completed all twelve weeks of the program, but because of a family emergency was not able to stick to it as diligently as she would have liked. Still, she was able to make exercise and healthy eating a habit, getting up an hour before work to exercise as often as she could with her busy schedule, usually two or three days a week instead of the four or five she had originally planned. Sometimes she felt as if she was failing at her goal, but then she realized she had set the bar too high and instead was glad she could work out as much as she did instead of beating herself up for not working out more.

Margie mastered the Level I circuits in six weeks and spent the next six weeks in Level II. She unexpectedly found that exercise was an excellent stress reliever at a time when she desperately needed to destress. Even though she was extra busy, Margie made time for herself and lost 7 pounds in the process, just short of her initial goal of 10. She and her family took the trip to Hawaii, and though she didn't wear a bikini, Margie enjoyed her new-found strength and athleticism and actually took a surfing lesson with her kids, something she never thought she could do!

Her New Goal
"In the next twelve weeks I will master the Level II moves and will get to work on Level III—they look hard but I am excited to try them! I will stick to my early-morning workouts three to four days a week, will lose another 7 pounds through consistent exercise and healthy eating, and will finally wear a bikini at the pool when the kids have swimming lessons!"

Sally

Her Original Goal
"I will lose 10 to 12 pounds in three months by exercising four days a week. I will cook more healthy meals for myself and my fiancé so that by my wedding date (in three months and one week!), I will fit into my original size 8 wedding dress and won't have to pay for massive alterations!"

Her Story
Since Sally works at home, she was able to exercise four days a week as she had planned. She mastered the Level I moves in four weeks and the Level II moves in six weeks. She spent the last two weeks of her twelve-week program doing the Level III moves. Sometimes she even got in an extra cardio workout when she was feeling energetic. She discovered she really liked running—it energized her while also helping clear her head. Sally bought some healthy cookbooks and prepared healthy meals for herself and her fiancé on a consistent basis. Because of her influence, he also started running and they often worked out together.

Through diligent workout planning and consistent healthful eating, Sally successfully lost the 12 pounds she intended to lose, but she still had to pay for dress alterations—she was smaller than a size 8! Her new, athletic body was more compact, so she had to have her dress taken in rather than let out, and she felt wonderful! Her new husband and she joined a local running club together and are planning on running a few races.

Her New Goal
"In two months I will train for and run a 5K. I will circuit train three days a week using the Level II and Level III moves to increase my strength and endurance and maintain my new fit body. I will also incorporate one dedicated day of flexibility training into my plan to help prevent injury. I also aim to lose another 5 pounds."

Kate

Her Original Goal
"In the next twelve weeks, I will eat healthy and exercise regularly to get my diabetes under control. I intend to be medication free by this time next year."

Her Story
Kate began a fitness program because she was diagnosed with diabetes and was put on medication. She hated the idea of spending a lifetime on meds, so she took the initiative to get into shape. She cleaned up her diet according to her doctor's recommendations and followed a sensible, healthy eating plan to get her blood sugar under control according to the *Your Body, Your Life* guidelines. This in itself was hard for Kate, who ate a lot of fast food and loved desserts. She had few weak moments when she lost her resolve and went to the drive-through, but instead of berating

herself and stewing over this minor setback, she kept her eye on her goal and got right back to healthy eating the next day.

The first four weeks of the workout program were extremely hard for Kate, who was obese, and she struggled with the Level I workouts. She could barely get through all the moves and was constantly sore, tired, and depressed. But before long, she was able to do all the moves in the Level I workouts, and by the end of twelve weeks was able to complete each Level I circuit without stopping. As she progressed, she began to lose weight, and she had lost a grand total of 18 pounds at the end of twelve weeks. She was elated! Moreover, her dependency on medication was drastically reduced, and her doctor was very hopeful that she would eventually be medication free.

Her New Goal

"In the next twelve weeks I will perfect the Level I moves and will move on to the Level II workouts. I will lose another 10 pounds and will again try to cut down my dependency on diabetes medication, moving toward my goal of being med free in nine more months. I will continue my healthy eating plan and will take a cooking class so I can learn to make foods that will improve my health."

Did you learn anything from reading these individual stories? While all three of these women have drastically different situations, they all formulated preliminary goals that were, for the most part, realistic and achievable. When they had a setback, they took it in stride and made adjustments instead of giving up completely. When they had completed their initial twelve weeks, they used their experience to help formulate their next set of goals.

YOUR GOALS—AGAIN

Now it's time to review your own goals. Take out a blank sheet of paper or open to a new page in your journal and write your original goal at the top of the page. Underneath, write out how the last twelve weeks went physically and emotionally for you, including how far you got in the *Your Body, Your Life* workouts, how you did with your nutrition, and anything else relevant to your progress. Reviewing your journals can be a big help here, as they delineate patterns of eating and exercise you might not otherwise notice. If you've fallen short of a goal, review your journals carefully to determine the reason for your shortcoming.

To help review your progress, ask yourself these questions:

- **Did you accomplish your goal?** If your answer is yes, how did you go about doing that? If your answer is no, what set you back?
- **How do you feel about your progress?** Are you happy? Disappointed? Elated? Examine these emotions and determine why you are feeling them.
- **Did you experience any unforeseen incidences, such as a family emergency, an injury, or an increased workload?** What did you do to compensate for these incidences? How did they affect your progress?
- **Did you expect too much or too little of yourself?**
- **How far did you get in the *Your Body, Your Life* workout program?** Was your progress what you expected? What exercises or workouts were hard for you? What did you excel at? What do you need to work on?
- **Did anything surprise you—good or bad—about your results at the end**

of twelve weeks? Did you lose weight? Did you lose inches? Are you more fit? Do you have more energy?

- **How was your nutrition?** Did you stick to a healthy eating plan? If not, what happened? If so, how did you do it?
- **If you accomplished your initial goal, what will your next goal be?**
- **If you didn't accomplish your initial goal, how will you go about accomplishing it in the next twelve weeks?**
- **What will you do differently in the future to accomplish your goals?**

After answering these questions, use your answers to help you formulate new goals that will keep you progressing and moving forward in your quest for a fit and healthy lifestyle. This is only the beginning. There's nowhere to go but up!

SUMMARY

You should be so proud of yourself for completing twelve solid weeks of healthy living! But remember this is only the beginning, and living a healthy lifestyle takes work. But now that you've completed three whole months of living well and exercising consistently, I know you'll be able to make this a lifelong habit!

HOMEWORK

1. Write down ten words that describe how you feel about yourself, your body, and your personality today. Once you've written them all down, get out the original self-description list you made back in Week 1 (Chapter 6) and compare your results. See a difference? I bet you do!

2. Buy yourself two new journals for the next twelve weeks of your new, fit lifestyle! Write your new goal on the front page of your workout journal and decorate it if the mood strikes you.

3. For the next month, do some research online and try one new healthy recipe a week. Write your favorite ones in your food journal.

Extra Credit

1. Take another Polaroid of yourself and compare it to your original from Week 1. How do you look now compared to then? How do you feel about the person in each of those pictures? Write down ten words to describe each person. Compare these words to the words you used to describe that person in Week 1.

2. Pedometer revisited. If you bought a pedometer for Extra Credit in Chapter 4 and have not used it in a while, put it back on and count your steps again! I bet you're getting in twice as many as you did initially!

3. Get your body fat rechecked! Go to the same facility you went to in Week 1 and have yourself retested. Compare your results. I bet you done good, girlfriend!

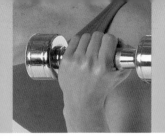

CHAPTER 18

Glitches and Gains

So did you sail through the first twelve weeks of your new fitness program with ease? Probably not! If you're like most people, you ran into some roadblocks. Be they personal, mental, physical, or uncontrollable, roadblocks are inevitable. How you react to them, however, is up to you. You can freak out about unforeseen setbacks, let your frustration get the best of you, and give up your intentions, or you can take these setbacks in stride, refuse to let them completely deter you, and get right back on track with your program.

In this chapter we'll cover some common roadblocks and offer some solutions for managing them with relative ease.

FAMILY/FRIEND SABOTAGE

While you probably expected your family and friends to support you in your decision to live a healthier lifestyle, you might have run into staunch resistance instead. This is not uncommon, and it probably made you feel horrible about your rela-

tionships with the individuals who opposed you. But know that their reactions are not your fault; people who are hostile as a result of your decision to change your lifestyle are simply scared to face their own issues with weight and health. Instead of coming to terms with their own problems, they choose to make you feel guilty and exposed. Often, they will try to sabotage your efforts at living a healthy lifestyle to make you more like them again, someone they understand and can relate to.

Don't let these people bring you down! A person who truly loves and respects you should support your decision to be healthier and happier. As heartbreaking as it may be, you might have to sever these destructive relationships. It would be great if these people could follow your lead instead of being so contrary, but you can't force them to change; they will change only when they are ready. You can, of course, maintain your healthy lifestyle and set an example for them to follow, but don't expect them to trot behind you willingly. They may choose to stay where they are while you move ahead mentally and physically into a better place. Instead of stressing about their resistance, nurture new relationships with healthy people who share your views and your attitude. These people will support you and your interests for years to come.

BINGEING

A lot of people first learning to eat healthfully restrict themselves excessively, building up a huge dam of craving that eventually bursts and leads to out-and-out bingeing. They eat anything and everything they get their hands on, and afterward they feel horrible—guilty, sick, and defeated. Often, they let these negative feelings take over, and they give up their program completely. If you've experienced a binge like this, you've got to overcome these negative feelings and move forward instead of letting them drag you back. Use these tips to help you overcome your issue:

- **Calculate your calories.** Cutting calories too low will often cause sugar cravings, which can ultimately lead to bingeing. Make sure you're getting enough calories to run your BMR and activities during the day. I never recommend cutting calories below 1,200 a day.

TALKING SENSE

Talk to your friends and family members in a noncombative way to defuse any misguided anger, jealousy, or hurt they may be feeling. See whether these phrases are useful to you when talking your loved ones off an angry ledge:

- I am choosing to live this healthy lifestyle to make my life better and make me feel better about myself. My decision was not consciously meant to make you feel angry or guilty about your own lifestyle.
- I do not think I am better than you; I am only trying to better myself.
- I do not love you any less because of my decision to change my own life.
- What I am doing is making me happier and healthier than I have been in years. I wish you could also be happy for me.
- Although I wish you would join me in my decision to life a healthier lifestyle, I will not judge you harshly if you choose not to.
- Even though I am living a healthier life, I am still the same person inside and still want us to be close.
- My life and my health are my responsibility; I am finally owning that responsibility.

- **Balance your nutrients.** Make sure you're eating the correct amounts of protein, carbs, and fat with all your meals. Often the body will crave something when it's missing certain nutrients, or if your meals don't "stick" with you very long. This usually occurs when you eat processed foods and high-glycemic carbs. Often adding a fat or protein to a meal

BINGE REBOUND, BY MARK

There is such a thing as eating too clean! I would never have believed it a year ago, but when you deprive yourself for so long, you're bound to reach a point where you go crazy. For instance, I had been eating squeaky clean for four months straight, and one night I broke down and ordered a pizza. I thought I would just have a couple of slices for a cheat meal, something Kim had recommended to me months ago (that I had yet to try) to keep cravings at bay. When the pizza came, I immediately ate two slices. It was so good! I didn't realize how much I had been craving that kind of food. Well, two slices turned into four, four turned to six, and all of a sudden I had eaten the whole pie! At first, I was devastated, guilty, and sick at the same time. But instead of letting this incident propel me into despair, I stepped back and thought: I have two choices. I can feel really bad about myself and go back to my old ways, or I can suck it up and move on. I realized I now had the tools with which to move forward, and that eating a whole pizza would not ruin my life. The next day I got right back to eating clean, and my body did not bear any ill effects of my food freak-out. After that, I started incorporating more regular cheat meals into my plan to avoid having a bingeing breakdown again.

increases its "stickability." Read your food journal and see where you may be lacking in certain macronutrients, adjusting your amounts to prevent cravings and bingeing.

- **Overdoing exercise?** Look through your workout journals to see whether you're exercising too much. Remember: An hour a day 4–6 days a week is plenty to make significant and lasting gains. More than this can lead to overtraining and burnout. It will also burn excessive calories, resulting in glycogen and blood sugar depletion and causing cravings.
- **Eat a cheat meal.** Having a cheat meal once a week can help alleviate cravings and keep you on track with your nutrition over the long haul. Once you get that craving out of your system, you'll be better able to focus on proper healthy nutrition for the rest of the week instead of obsessing about your craving.
- **Don't beat yourself up.** Everyone experiences temporary nutritional failures from time to time, even me! Though you may feel horrible and guilty about a binge session, try to take this setback in stride instead of berating yourself for it. Accept that it has happened, and get right back onto your healthy program as soon as possible to minimize the mental and physical damage that the bingeing may have caused.

INJURY

Injuries are unpredictable, and if you incur one, you might have to cut back on your workouts or even put them on hold while you heal. This forced hiatus might put you in an emotional funk, especially if you were really feeling good about yourself and your progress before sustaining the injury. But don't get frustrated and throw in the towel! Injuries don't have to completely debilitate you, and instead of giving up, there are several things you can do to maintain your gains while simultaneously rehabbing your injury quickly and safely.

- **Focus on nutrition.** While you're injured, eat as healthfully as possible. Cut back on simple carbs and focus on eating lots of lean protein and veggies. Also spend this downtime coming up with new recipes or reviewing your food journal to see where you can make improvements to your general plan.
- **Work on flexibility.** The healing of many injuries can be accelerated with consistent

stretching. Stretch your injured part gently and frequently according to your doctor's recommendations to regain your range of motion and ease stiffness and soreness. Also take this time to work on flexibility in other parts of your body that are tight and stiff to help prevent future injuries.

- **Remember the rule of relative rest.** While you do have to rest your injured part and allow it time to heal, you can still train other parts of your body. If you've sustained an upper-body injury, you can still do cardio and lower-body work; if you've sustained a lower-body injury, you can still work on your upper body and core strength and do light or moderate cardio according to your doctor's recommendations. Be creative and figure out ways to work around your injury instead of letting it sideline you completely.

BURNING QUESTION

I had bursitis in my shoulder, and I took the time off my doctor recommended. But three weeks after I started training again, it's back! What happened? You probably didn't give it enough time to heal, or you tried to go back to training too hard too soon. Doctors give you only a ballpark estimate of how long you should take off to heal an injury; sometimes it's enough time, sometimes it's not. It's up to you to gauge how your shoulder is feeling and whether or not it's ready to work. When you do start training again, start slowly; mentally you may be ready and raring to go, but physically your shoulder is back at square one. For a number of weeks, use lighter weights, fewer repetitions, and shorter circuit time increments. Also do lots of stretching and use RICE when you even think you feel a little

pain. Your body will tell you when it's ready to do more work. Just turn your ear inward and listen to what it's saying.

WORKOUT BOREDOM

Everyone experiences workout boredom, even me! Although I have tried my darndest to make the *Your Body, Your Life* circuits as interesting and challenging as possible, you're sure to get bored with them in time.

The first thing I recommend when faced with terminal boredom is a mini-vacation from exercise. Take a week completely off from training. Sometimes your brain needs a break from exercise as much as your body does, and a little downtime goes a long way toward recharging your mental intentions. After you've taken some time off, try rearranging your workouts to make them more inspiring and motivating, keeping your brain as motivated as your body. Check out these ideas:

- **Circuit Swap.** The circuits listed in this book are only suggested workouts. Once you're familiar with the moves and can do them all with good form, you can certainly change the order of the moves within the circuit, or change the order in which you do the circuits in the course of the week. You can even combine moves from different levels to make your own circuit! Be creative and change things around constantly to keep your brain and body guessing.
- **Body-Part Blast.** Tailor your circuit workouts to hit specific body parts you'd like to improve. If you want more definition in your arms, for example, assemble an all-upper-body workout from the moves you've mastered. Do this workout twice a week and your lower-body/

SAMPLE BODY-PART BLAST

UPPER-BODY CIRCUIT (LEVEL II MOVES)

- Bi-Row
- Uptown Arms
- Back to Business
- Fly Like an Eagle
- Tough-Girl Push-ups
- Shoulder T
- Kick 'n' Row
- Fly-Girl Curls
- Circle T
- Superman

cardio workouts twice a week; you'll still be hitting all your body parts, just in a different way.

NUTRITION BOREDOM

Good nutrition isn't always exciting, and you may burn out on egg whites and oatmeal after a while. This is normal, and again, sometimes all you need is a week off to mentally recharge your intentions. But I bet you won't make it a whole week! In fact, you'll probably find it hard to stray from your new way of eating for more than a few days. I know it sounds crazy, but eating healthfully makes you feel so good mentally and physically that you'll notice an immediate difference in your energy when you go back to making poor nutritional choices. After taking some time off, try a few of these tips to make your nutrition more interesting.

- **Spice it up.** Try new herbs and spices in your favorite dishes and see how they turn out. For instance, do you know what to do with cardamom? Me neither, but I bet there are tons of recipes out there that use it, and they are probably fabulous! Look up cardamom and other spices you haven't tried before online or in cookbooks, and see which foods they compliment and how to use them properly.

- **Use the Net.** You can find any recipe you can imagine online! Just now, I tried typing "fat-free strawberry shortcake" into my search engine and came up with more than 200,000 results! Investigate new recipes or search for healthy modifications of your favorite dishes. Also check out the thousands of online blogs, cooking Web sites, and personal recipe pages available in cyberspace. Sign up for some free recipe and cooking newsletters and your idea coffer will overflow in no time!

- **Learn from a master.** Cooking classes can reinspire you to be creative with your nutrition and can also connect you to people of similar interests. Food and friends—what more could you ask for? The price for these classes runs the gamut, from expensive celebrity chef seminars to economical cooking classes held at community colleges and recreational centers around the country. Check your local paper to see what is available in your area.

- **Go out to eat.** You can find tons of restaurants that offer healthy menu items if you look carefully and order wisely. My favorite healthy dining places are sushi bars, seafood restaurants, and any other establishments that are willing to cook things to order. Remember to have everything grilled, steamed, or broiled, order all the sauces and condiments on the side, and forego the bread, heavy alcohol, and dessert!

HOLIDAYS AND SPECIAL EVENTS

Everyone frets about gaining weight over the holidays or at special events, and truthfully I could write an entire book just on managing your weight and your stress during these times! But you can still enjoy your holidays and events without compromising your healthy plan by following these tips:

- **Be pot-lucky.** If you're invited to a potluck party, bring several of your own favorite low-fat dishes. Stick to eating these during the party, no matter how tempting the others might be!
- **Be a healthy host.** When hosting a party or event, cook all your dishes in a healthy way, even birthday cakes! Chances are your guests won't even know the difference.
- **Pull a party pre-eat.** Never go to a party hungry! Always eat a healthy meal about an hour before arriving to avoid pigging out on things you wouldn't otherwise eat. I have been known to eat a Ziploc baggie of tuna and rice in the car right before hitting a holiday party! It sounds weird, but it keeps me from chowing on high-fat nibbles and snacks.
- **Abridge alcohol.** Alcohol and resolve have an inverse relationship: The more alcohol you consume, the less you resolve to stick to your nutrition guns! Keep your tippling to a minimum, not only because of the high calorie content of alcoholic beverages, but also to stay mentally on track with your healthy plan.
- **Up your H$_2$O.** For every alcoholic beverage you drink, also consume one full glass of water. This will cut the effects of the alcohol while filling your stomach, making you less likely to indulge.
- **Indulge, but don't overindulge.** Sometimes you simply want to enjoy party food, and that's OK. Just do it in moderation. Take a small taste—one or two bites at the most—of everything that looks good. If you absolutely love it, have a little bit more. If you don't love it, don't finish it. Why waste calories on so-so

snacks and sweets? If you're gonna go overboard, make it worth the swim!
- **Keep exercising.** To minimize party-food damage and ward off stress, maintain your exercise program. You probably won't lose any weight if you're attending a lot of food-related events, but you can certainly maintain the fitness level you've already established, making it that much easier to get on track once the holidays are over.

PREGNANCY

Many women get pregnant while trying to establish a fit and healthy lifestyle, but being pregnant is not an excuse to pig out! Take my contestant Heather from Season 3 of *The Biggest Loser*. Shortly after returning home from the ranch, Heather got pregnant with her second child. But instead of

PERIODIZE TO PROGRESS

Athletes periodize their training to maximize results while minimizing injury potential. You, too, can use this system to your advantage to keep your body progressing and keep boredom at bay. A simple periodization program might look like this: Using the Level I circuits, map out a three-week schedule. For all your workouts the first week, use lighter weights and do the exercise for a longer time with shorter rest in between moves. For all your workouts the second week, use moderate weights and moderate work and rest intervals. And for all your workouts the third week, use heavy weights, shorter work intervals, and longer rest periods. Because of the varying weights and time increments, your body gets a different stimulus every week, even when you're using the same circuits.

SAMPLE WORKOUT SCHEDULE: LEVEL I CIRCUITS
Week 1: 5-pound dumbbells, 1 minute per move, 30 seconds of rest
Week 2: 8-pound dumbbells, 45 seconds per move, 45 seconds of rest
Week 3: 10-pound dumbbells, 30 seconds per move, 1 minute of rest
Week 4: Repeat Week 1

CHANGE YOUR CARDIO

If you always do the same cardio routine, you're bound to get bored. Shake things up a little from week to week, changing your modality often to keep from burning out. For instance, last month I was really into running stairs, while this month I am totally dedicated to in-line skating. I change things around all the time to keep both my brain and my body entertained!

SOME GREAT ALTERNATIVE CARDIO IDEAS
- Buy a local trail map and go hiking.
- Go to a track and run sprints.
- Find a set of stadium stairs and do drills.
- Try a new sport such snowboarding, skiing, wakeboarding, or surfing.
- Use a free day pass at a local gym to try Spinning, Pilates, yoga, Step, or another group class.
- Change your walking, jogging, or biking route every other week.
- Try a new machine at the gym, even if it looks scary! It might turn out to be your favorite.

abandoning her program and going back to her old ways, she stuck to it, even through severe morning sickness and a sharp decline in appetite. She appeared on TV at five months pregnant looking healthy and fit instead of bloated and overstuffed.

Here are some tips for staying healthy and fit while you're pregnant:

• **Consult your physician.** Tell your doctor of your plan to maintain your nutrition and exercise routine during your pregnancy. Chances are your doctor will encourage you to do so! However, women with risky pregnancies should absolutely follow the advice of their doctors to the letter; if your doctor tells you not to work out, listen! No fitness plan is worth risking the life of your baby!

• **Modify your activity.** Your heart rate when you're pregnant is naturally higher than normal, so use the RPE scale (see page 56) when gauging intensity. If you're using a heart rate monitor, try to keep your heart rate below 140 when exercising, and avoid supine (on your back) activity, such as abdominal exercises, after the first trimester. You also become more flexible when you're pregnant, so be careful not to overstretch yourself when practicing flexibility.

• **Eat *healthy* for two.** The old adage of "eating for two" is completely outdated! Research indicates that you need only 300 additional calories a day to produce a healthy, happy baby, so being pregnant is not an excuse to stuff yourself with junk foods and sweets. Excess calories you take in while pregnant (minus the 300 a day for baby growing) will still be stored as fat! To avoid excess weight gain, choose healthy foods to get in those extra 300 baby-growing calories, such as fresh fruit, lean meats, lots of veggies, and the occasional sweet treat.

• **Indulge your cravings—sometimes.** Just because you're craving an ice-cream-and-pickle sandwich at bedtime doesn't mean you should eat it! Cravings are more mental than anything, so try to satisfy them with a healthy substitution. Try a low-fat pudding snack or a Wasa cracker with peanut butter and see whether your craving dissipates. If it doesn't, give in to the ice-cream-and-pickle sandwich—just make it a small one!

SUMMARY

The road to wellness is rife with roadblocks. Whether your roadblock comes in the form of holidays, family strife, bingeing, injury, or boredom, you now have all the tools to manage them with a level head and common sense. Whatever obstacles you come across, manage them calmly, accept their occurrence, and move forward with confidence.

HOMEWORK

1. Go to a restaurant for dinner this week. Practice the tips listed in the "Eating Out" sidebar for a more healthful dining experience.

2. Create your own workout circuit! Use the moves from whatever level you're comfortable with and arrange them in a new way.

3. This month, do something different every week for cardio. Use the suggestions on page 254 for ideas.

4. Buy a cooking magazine or do an online search and try two new healthy recipes this month.

5. Make a list of all things that you think are "out of your control" and resolve to improve the situation.

Extra Credit

Look up these spices and use them in healthy dishes this month:

- coriander
- cayenne pepper
- cilantro
- turmeric
- paprika
- curry powder
- mint
- basil

EATING OUT

Eating out is not evil! Follow these tips for the healthiest—and still enjoyable—dining experience possible.

- Ask your server not to bring bread and butter before your meal. Why tempt fate?
- If you're having an alcoholic beverage, skip the starch in your entrée and ask for steamed vegetables instead.
- Ask to have any sauces, condiments, or dressings put on the side instead of on top of your food. That way, you—not the chef—have complete control over how much you add.
- Ask to substitute a salad for a starchy side. Usually restaurants will do this for a small charge.
- Ask that your food be prepared with no oil, butter, or added salt.
- Leave off the cheese on salads, appetizers, and entrees, and save up to 300 calories!
- Opt for vegetable- and tomato-based soups and sauces instead of cream- and cheese-based ones.
- Read the menu carefully to see whether the restaurant offers any healthy or dieter's options.
- Ask to have your entrée broiled or grilled instead of sautéed or fried. This will greatly reduce the fat calories added to your food while cooking.
- Ask for a to-go box to come with your entrée. Immediately put half of your dinner into the box and put it away. If it's not on your plate, you're less likely to eat it, and you'll have a great lunch tomorrow!
- If you're having a dessert, go for the lower-calorie options such as sorbet or fruit. Better yet, share one dessert with the whole table! One piece of cake split into six pieces will give each person fewer calories than one dish of sorbet eaten alone.
- And finally the Golden Rule: If your food does not come out as ordered, send it back. Don't "settle" for what you've been given if it's not right. You're paying for it, you're going to be eating it, and it should be made correctly. Simply send it back—*politely*—and have the kitchen remake your meal to your specifications.

CHAPTER 19

Maintaining Motivation

To make health and fitness a lifestyle, staying motivated is key. This is the hardest part about the whole process! Motivation is a very personal thing, and what motivates one person might not do it for another. The trick is to find what motivates you personally, and run with it! Here are some suggestions to help you find some motivation when the going gets tough and your inspiration is flagging.

- **Reset your goals.** Goal setting is a highly motivating practice. If you've already reached a goal and are feeling lost and aimless, set another one! Use the goals you've already accomplished to help guide you in the process of making new goals. Remember to make all goals realistic and attainable so that you are able to reach them and stay motivated and upbeat instead of discouraged and unsuccessful.
- **Remake your mantras.** Revisit and rework your mantras to suit your new goals. If you haven't been using a mantra, try it out! You might be surprised at how well they work.
- **Pause at the poster.** Take a few minutes and stand in front of your goal poster, remembering why you made it and noticing how far you've come. If you haven't yet reached it, remember your end goal, and fire yourself up to get there. If you've already reached your end goal, make a new poster! But don't toss your first one. Old goal posters can remind you of how far you've come, giving you a little extra spark to reignite your motivation.
- **Buddy up.** Working out with a friend or family member is a great way to stay motivated. You can encourage each other and make each other accountable for your actions. See whether one of your friends, neighbors, or family members would like to buddy up and share your healthy new lifestyle. If you can't find a live workout buddy, there are tons of cyberspace buddies to be had. The Internet offers chat rooms, blogs, even whole Web sites dedicated to helping you

stay motivated and continue with your new healthy lifestyle. Some of them cost a bit of money, but for a few dollars a week you can have access to thousands of people just like you who are having the same trials and successes you're having.

BURNING QUESTION

What about Weight Watchers, Overeaters Anonymous, and other such support-group meetings—are they good for motivation? Of course! Anything that allows you to express your joys and frustrations with others experiencing the same things can be a great motivator. But be sure the meetings you're attending are productive and uplifting rather than discouraging and gloomy. Don't allow yourself to get dragged down by those who are negative and unhappy, dedicated to wallowing in self-pity and depression. You can certainly try to buoy them up, encouraging them and motivating them to be healthy and happy, but if those in your meetings continually drag you down, find a different meeting—there are tons of them out there. If you can't find one that suits you, start your own!

- **Find a league of your own.** Many recreational or community centers have a schedule of adult sports lessons and leagues, offering classes in activities such as golf, tennis, volleyball, softball, flag football, and cycling. Most offer beginning classes as well as advanced ones, so it doesn't matter if you've never played before.

- **Join a gym.** While some of you may be perfectly comfortable training at home, others might benefit from joining a gym. Gyms offer a wide range of equipment, machines, and classes that can help inspire and motivate you. If you're not comfortable in a large coed facility, look for an all-women's gym or a center with a women-only weight room. Visit a few gyms to see which ones appeal to you. Most offer a free week trial membership, so you can test-drive the facility to see whether it suits your needs.

- **Peruse the periodicals.** There are tons and tons of great health and fitness magazines out there just waiting to inspire you! These monthly publications offer great workout ideas, new recipes, personal stories, and even motivational tips! Go to the bookstore or library and browse a bit. Buy a few you think you might like, then subscribe to those that really inspire and motivate you. Some of my favorites are *Self, Women's Health, Oxygen,* and *Muscle and Fitness.*

- **Be a bookworm.** Books can be as inspiring and motivating as magazines. For instance, even though I am not a cyclist, I love all of Lance Armstrong's books! All I have to do is read one of his books, and any problem I am having pales in comparison—I mean, the man beat stage 4 cancer to win the Tour de France seven times! Nothing is more inspiring to me than reading a story like that.

- **Have a fat-jeans fashion show.** Many clients of mine have kept a piece of clothing that represents them at their heaviest weight. When they're feeling down and need some instant inspiration, they take out that item of clothing and try it on. It reminds them of how far they have come and helps them focus again on their intentions.

EXERCISE YOUR INFLUENCE

Another way to stay inspired is to inspire others! Share your newfound knowledge with those in your family and community so that they, too, can experience the incredible lifestyle you've discovered. You're now a fitness expert in your own right, and it's time to pay it forward.

- **Walk this way.** What better way to give to your community and to yourself than by starting a walking club! It can be as official or unofficial as you'd like, single-sex or coed, limited to friends and family or encompassing an entire apartment complex. It's your group—make it what you'd like! If you're a big thinker, advertise your group in your local or community paper, or in your homeowners' newsletter, extending your reach beyond your immediate circle of peers.
- **Be charitable.** Organize a running race, a baseball game, a potato-sack race, or even a rodeo to benefit charity. Use your imagination and get creative—there are so many ways to be active, and any event that gets people moving is a great idea! Charge a small entry fee for participants to help fund it, and donate the extra proceeds to your favorite charity.

- **Get to your grocer.** Solicit your deli owner, butcher, and grocer to stock healthier items in their stores. Have specific items in mind that you'd like them to carry, such as organic produce, trans-fat-free bakery items, and whole-grain goods and products. Suggest healthier cuts of meat or request new kinds of fish and seafood at the butcher's station.
- **Be a healthy host.** Host a cookout, party, or event where you make nothing but healthy fare, or organize a potluck in which all guests must bring a healthy item. Have everyone write their recipes and e-mail addresses on index cards; then, when the party is over, compile the recipes and send them out to all who attended!
- **Be pro-active parents.** America's kids are fat, and it's up to you to help solve this problem. Set a healthy example for your kids now! Plan active outings with your family—take a family hike, take long walks together after dinner, or a go on a weekend skiing and sledding adventure. Anything that involves togetherness and activity is a good bet. Limit the time your kids spend in front of the TV playing sports video games, and instead get them outside to play actual sports!
- **Those who can, do teach!** Some of my most successful clients have been so inspired by their own journeys that they have gone on to become certified personal trainers, aerobics instructors, sports coaches, and even fitness competitors! They want to inspire those around them to live a healthier, happier life through fitness and have chosen a career path that allows them to do just that.
- **Speak out.** Many of my successful clients find enormous satisfaction speaking to groups, companies, and schools about their experiences with weight loss. They are able to connect to those experiencing

the same things they did when they were at their heaviest, and are able to relate to them on a personal level, inspiring and motivating those who are despairing to get up and do something about it.

MOVING WORDS

If you're still in need of motivation, here are some inspiring words from some terrific clients of mine!

When I got back from the Biggest Loser ranch, a lot of my friends wanted to lose weight, too, so I wrote up a few pages about what I did. Now almost all of my friends have been exercising and losing weight! Even my niece, a freshman in high school who is 200 pounds and on blood pressure meds because of her weight, started using my tips and has already gone down a pants size in three weeks! It's amazing to be able to help people like that. —Pam

After I lost a ton of weight with Kim, a lady who watched The Biggest Loser *actually called and joined my gym because I inspired her! When the assistant manager told me this, I asked when she was coming in so I could be there. Why not? I inspired someone to come to the gym and lose weight, and I wanted to be there in person to give her the motivation she needed to continue! That is my whole thing now. I want to take a vested interest in the people around me and help them do what I was able to do.* —Ken

People who see what I accomplished with Kim on TV approach me and say, "You inspired me to lose weight," or "You inspired me to stop smoking," or "You inspired my dad who just had a heart attack to start exercising." It's an honor and a privilege to be given the opportunity to change my life

and also to help others. What an amazing gift. —Mark

I lost 50 pounds and got rid of my asthma and chronic back pain through walking and working with Kim. When my mother saw how much my life had changed, she started walking with me twice a week in the hopes of losing a bit of weight. After a few weeks, she felt pretty good and started walking with me four days a week. Six months later, she had lost 20 pounds! She was so inspired she started a walking club with her church group. —Paula

SUMMARY

If you're as excited as I am about your progress, you'll want to share your "secrets of success" with others! Be a proactive member of your community, planning healthy activities and offering help and encouragement to those who need it most. Sharing your knowledge with others is often as rewarding as learning it yourself.

HOMEWORK

1. Have a healthy dinner party. Invite friends and family over for a good, nutritious meal.
2. Ask a friend or family member to start exercising with you.
3. Go to your local gym and check it out.
4. Write down five things that motivate you to be healthy and active. See how this list compares to the one you made back in Chapter 2.

Extra Credit

Have an active birthday party event for your kids! Instead of sitting around watching movies and eating chips, take the party outside to your local park. Organize a baseball game, have potato-sack races, or even host a scavenger hunt.

Epilogue

I have been talking about writing a book like this for nearly a decade, and I am so thankful to finally have been given the forum in which to share my knowledge and experience about something I love so dearly. Nothing is more inspiring to me than seeing someone use the simple tools I give them to change their lives completely! I am continually amazed at what the human body and mind can accomplish when the person inside is determined and strong.

I hope you've learned tons of new things in *Your Body, Your Life* and are so inspired by your results and experience that you continue with your new lifestyle for years to come. I also hope you don't stop here! I encourage you to read more, learn more, and share what you know with others. Nothing is more beautiful than the gift of health, and if each person who reads this book shares his or her knowledge with one other person, we can fight the obesity epidemic one life at a time.

So while this book has come to its conclusion, your journey has not. It's simply *Ciao for now!* I know our paths will cross again soon!

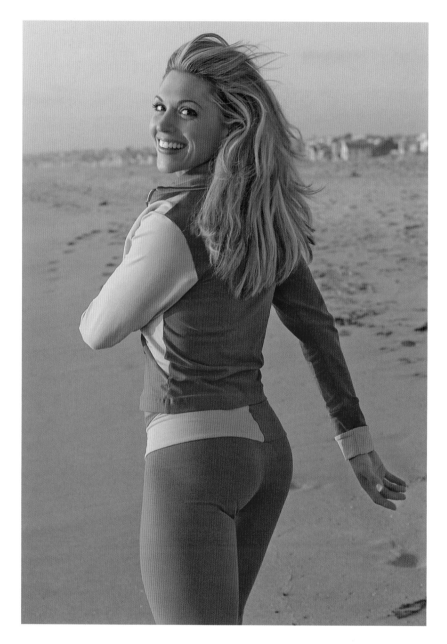

INDEX

Ab Cycle, 83
Abductor Lift, 108
Activities, trying different, 22–23
Acute injuries, 175
Advanced Superman, 140
Alcohol, 201–203
Appetite suppressants, 188
Athletic shoes, 2, 178

Back to Business (Bent-Over Row / Rear Shoulder Fly), 98
Balance Test, 40
Balancing Biceps (Single Leg Squat / Biceps Curl), 128
Balancing Booty Burner (Reverse Lunge / Glute Raise and Balance / Rear Shoulder Fly), 133
Balancing Booty Burner (Reverse Lunge / Glute Raise / Bent-Over Row), 134
Ballet Squat, 74
Ballet Squat Plus (Ballet Squat / Calf Raise), 105
Ballet Super-Squat Combo (Ballet Squat / Calf Raise / Upright Row), 135
Basal metabolic rate (BMR), 10, 211
Basic Crunch, 82
Basic March, 87
Basic Reverse Lunge, 71
Basic Squat, 73
Basic Squat / Close Squat, 107
Basic Squat / Inner Thigh, 103
Beers, low-carb, 203
Beginner workout moves, 59–93
Beginning Burpee, 92
Beginning Power Lunge, 89
Beginning Side Lunge, 72
Beginning Superman, 77
Bent-Over Row, 84, 109, 134, 138
Bent-Over Row / Rear Shoulder Fly, 98
Biceps Curl, 63, 128
Biceps Curl / Upright Row / Glute Raise, 127
Biceps Strongman Curl / Straight-Arm Chest Fly, 100
Biggest Loser, The, iv
Bingeing, 249–250
Bioelectrical impedance analysis (BIA), 11
Bi-Row (Biceps Curl / Upright Row), 95
Body
  appreciating, 5
  composition of, 10–11
  inner workings of, 5–14
  responsibility for, 13–14
Body fat percentage, determining, 11
Body measurements, 36
Body-Part Blast, 251–252
Body type, 6–7
Breakfast, 210
  recipes for, 224–227
Breathing, 62
Bridge, 116
Bridge Bonus, 142
Bulk cooking, 218–219
Bunny Hop, 90

Burpee, 124, 177
  Beginning, 92
  Power, 157
Butt-Bi-Row (Biceps Curl / Upright Row / Glute Raise), 127
Butterfly Stretch, 171

Calf Raise, 105, 135
Calf Stretch, 159
Calorie-burning activities, 26
Calorie-restrictive diets, 186–187
Calories, counting, 210–211, 249
Calorie schedules, 211–212
Carbohydrates, 191–194
  portion sizes for, 207–208
Cardio Rx
  Level I, 62
  Level II, 94
  Level III, 126
Cardiovascular training, 46, 48, 49, 54, 55
  rules for, 57
Cat/Dog, 169
Cheat meals, 213, 250
Chest Fly
  90-Degree, 69, 99, 132
  Straight-Arm, 100, 102
Chest Stretch, 165
Circle T, 101
Circuit swap, 251
Circuit training, 50–51, 58
  rules for, 56–57
  system, viii
Close Squat, 75
Clothing, 3–4
  appropriate, 179
Comfort zone, 15–16
Complete proteins, 191
Complex carbohydrates, 192
Compliment journal, 8
Compression, for injuries, 176
Cooking. See Meal planning; Recipes
Cool-down, 179
"Crash" dieting, 186–187
Cravings, 200, 244, 254
Cross trainers, 2
Cross-training, 175–176, 181
Crouching Stretch, 166
Crunch
  Basic, 82
  Feet-Up, 117
  Punch, 144
  Reach-for-the-Sky, 143
Crunch Test, 38
Curl
  Biceps, 63, 127
  Strongman, 64

Daily activity, increasing, 195
Daily goals, 25
Deadlift, 138
Delayed-onset muscle soreness (DOMS), 179
Dessert recipes, 237–239
Detours, managing, 30–31, 33
Diabetes, 13
Dieter's teas, 187–188
Dinner recipes, 233–236
Donkey Kick, 79
  Straight-Leg, 113

Donkey Kick Bonus, 145
  Straight-Leg, 146
Double-Duty Delts, 97
"Double moves," 94
Dumbbells, 2

Ectomorphs, 7
Elevation, for injuries, 176
Elimination diets, 185–186
Emotional eating, 16–17, 31
Endomorphs, 7
Endorphins, 49–50
"Essential fat," 10

Fad diets, 184–189
  types of, 185–188
Family, as supporters, 22
Fat-free foods, 200–201
Fats
  dietary, 194–195
  portion sizes for, 207
"Feeling the work," 60
Feet-Up Crunch, 117
Fiber, 196–197
Finger-Touch Test, 39
Fitness, 35–43
  reevaluating, 242–247
Fitness magazines, 257–258
Fitness program
  roadblocks in, 248–255
  starting, 1
Fitness tests, 37–40
  retaking, 242–243
Fitness triangle, 48–50, 51
Flat-back posture, 9
Flexibility training, 47, 49, 51, 55, 159
Floor Punch, 130
Fly-Girl Curls (Biceps Strongman Curl / Straight-Arm Chest Fly), 100
Fly Like an Eagle (Overhead Shoulder Press / 90-Degree Chest Fly), 99
Food basics, 190
Food journals, 31–34
Food labels, reading, 219–221
Food notes, 32
Foods, high-quality, 183
Food shopping list, 216–217
"Free" foods, 200–201
Front Shoulder Raise, 70
Front Shoulder Raise / Lateral Shoulder Raise, 97
Front Shoulder Raise / Straight-Arm Chest Fly, 102
Full Jack, 121
Full Power Lunge, 149
Future fitness, planning for, 241–261

Gear, 2–4
Genetic health problems, 11
Genetics, 6
Get Hip (Side-Lying Leg Lift / Side-Lying Knee to Chest), 115
Get-real questions, 21–22
Girly Push-up, 76
Glute Raise, 127, 129, 130, 133, 134
Glute Stretch, 172
Glycemic index (GI), 192, 193
Goal poster, 24
Goal review, 244–247

Goals, 21–28
  activity-related, 26, 27
  long-term, 23–24
  realistic, 27
  resetting, 256
  short-term, 24–25
Good habits, creating, 17–18
Grocery shopping, 214–217
Gym, joining, 257

Habits. *See also* Good habits
  choosing, 17
  making and breaking, 16–17
Half Jack, 86
Half Plank, 78
Half Power Lunge, 118
Hamstring Curl, 129
Hamstring Stretch, 170
Health, 11–13
Health problems, 23
Heart disease, 12
Heart rate monitors, 56
Heat, for injuries, 176
Hidden sugar, 200
High blood pressure, 12–13, 14, 203, 204–205
High-Knee Reverse Lunge, 104
High-Knee Run, 151
Holidays, as roadblocks, 252–253
Hop Around the Clock, 150
Hydration, 197–199
Hypertension, 12–13, 14, 203, 204–205

Ice, for injuries, 176
Incomplete proteins, 191
Influence, exercising, 258–259
Injuries, 23
  preventing, 175, 179–181
  as roadblocks, 250–251
  types of, 175, 176–178
Insoluble fiber, 196
Inspiration, sharing, 258–260, 261
Intensity, measuring, 55

Journal review, 243–244
Journals, 4. *See also* Food journals; Workout journals
Jump Around the Clock, 120

Kick 'n' Row (Triceps Kickback / Bent-Over Row), 109
Kickback, Triceps, 85
Knee Raise, 106
Knees-Up March, 123
Knee to Chest, Side-Lying, 81, 115
Kung Fu Reverse Lunge, 131

Lateral Shoulder Raise, 68
Laxatives, 187
Lean mass, 10–11
Leg Lift, Side-Lying, 80, 115
Leg Squat, Single, 128
Level I workout moves, 63–93
Level II workout moves, 94–125
Level III workout moves, 126–158
Lordosis posture, 9
Low-carb diet, 185–186
Lower-Body / Cardio Workouts, 52, 55
Low Flow (Triceps Kickback / Step Out / Punch), 137

Lunch recipes, 227–231
Lunge
  Basic Reverse, 71
  Beginning Power, 89
  Beginning Side, 72
  Full Power, 149
  Half Power, 118
  High-Knee Reverse, 104
  Kung Fu Reverse, 131
  Reverse, 133, 134
  Runner's, 167
  Side, 108, 130
Lyons, Kim, iv–v
Mantras, 19–20
  remaking, 256
March
  Basic, 87
  Knees-Up, 123
Maximum heart rate (MHR), 57
Meal-replacement shakes, 186
Meals, 206–213
  planning of, 218–221
  timing of, 208–210
Measurements, taking, 36
Medi-alerts, 179
Mental barriers, identifying, 20
Mesomorphs, 7
Metabolism, 10
  fueling, 209–210
Mirror, full-length, 3
Mogul Jump, 153
Monthly goals, 25
Motivation, maintaining, 256–260
Motives, questioning, 16
Mountain Climber, 148
Muscles
  locations of, 60–61
  soreness in, 179
  toning, 48
Music, 46

National Academy of Sports Medicine
  (NASM), v
Neck Stretch, 168
Negative self-talk, 18–19
90-Degree Chest Fly, 69, 99, 132
"No-sugar-added" products, 221
Nutrition, 183–189
  balanced, 185, 249–250
Nutrition boredom, 252

Obesity, 12
Open and Close Squat (Basic Squat /
  Close Squat), 107
Overhead Front Raise / Overhead Triceps
  Extension, 96
Overhead Shoulder Press, 67
Overhead Shoulder Press / 90-Degree
  Chest Fly, 99
Overhead Triceps Extension, 65
Overtraining, 54–55, 244
Overuse injuries, 175, 176

Pain, 179
Pedometers, 26, 28
Physical limitations, 23
Physicals, 14
Pilates, 50

Plank, 112
  Side, 114
  Windmill, 147
Plank Plus, 141
Plyo Squat, 152, 156
Pop Squat, 156
Portion sizes, 206–208
Positive speech, 19
Posture, 8–9
Potassium, 203
Power Burpee, 157
Power Lunge, Beginning, 89
Pregnancy, 253–254
Protein, 190–191
  portion sizes for, 207
Protein drinks, 186
Pulled muscles, 178
Punch Crunch, 144
Push-up
  Girly, 76
  Split-Hand, 139
  Tough-Girl, 110
Push-up Test, 37

Quad Stretch, 160

Rate of perceived exertion (RPE)
  scale, 55, 56
Reach-for-the-Sky Crunch, 143
Recipes, 222–239
Relative rest, ice, compression, and
  elevation (RICE), 176
Relative rest rule, 251
Resistance training, 10, 47, 48
Rest, for injuries, 176
Rest days, 54–55, 181
Reverse Lunge, Basic, 71
Rewards, 27, 242–243
Row
  Bent-Over, 84, 138
  Upright, 66, 127, 135
Run, High-Knee, 151
Runner's Lunge, 167

Sabotage, by family or friends, 248–249
Safety equipment, 179
Saturated fats, 194
Scoliosis, 10
Seesaw (Deadlift / Bent-Over Row /
  Rear Shoulder Fly), 138
Self-criticism, 20
Self-esteem, low, 18
Self-talk, negative, 18–19
Shin splints, 177
Shoes, appropriate, 179
Shoulder Fly, 98
  Rear, 133, 138
Shoulder Press, Overhead, 67, 129,
  132
Shoulder Raise, 97
  Front, 70, 130
  Lateral, 68
Shoulder Stretch, 163
Shoulder T (Front Shoulder Raise /
  Straight-Arm Chest Fly), 102
Side dish recipes, 231–233
Side Lunge, Beginning, 89
Side Lunge 'n' Lift (Side Lunge /

Abductor Lift), 108
Side Lunge 'n' Lift 'n' Lift (Side Lunge /
  Floor Punch / Front Shoulder Raise /
  Glute Raise), 130
Side-Lying Knee to Chest, 81
Side-Lying Leg Lift, 80
Side-Lying Leg Lift / Side-Lying Knee
  to Chest, 115
Side Plank, 114
Side Stretch, 161
Simple carbohydrates, 192
Single Leg Squat / Biceps Curl, 128
Sit-and-Reach Test, 39
Skeletal structure, 8
Ski Hop, 119
Skin-fold testing, 11
Sleep quality, 181
Snacks, 208–209
  for kids, 214–215
  recipes for, 223–224
Soccer Squat (Basic Squat / Inner
  Thigh), 103
Socks, 4
Sodium, 203–204
Soluble fiber, 196
Speed Skate, 122
  Starter, 91
  Super, 155
Spinal Twist, 173
Split-Hand Push-up, 139
Sports bra, 4
Sports drinks, 198–199
Spot-reducing, 7–8
Spouse, as a supporter, 22
Sprains, 177–178
Squat
  Ballet, 74, 105, 135
  Basic, 73
  Close, 75, 132
  Open and Close, 107
  Plyo, 152
  Pop, 156
  Single Leg, 128
  Soccer, 103
  Super, 132
Squat Plus (Close Squat / Knee Raise),
  106
Squat Test, 38
Starter Speed Skate, 91
"Starvation mode," 26
Steam Engine, 136
Step Touch, 88
Straight-Leg Donkey Kick, 113
Straight-Leg Donkey Kick Bonus, 146
Strains, 178
Stress fracture, 178
Stretching
  moves, 159–174
  rules for, 57–58
Stretching routine, sample, 174
Strongman Curl, 64
Sugar, 199–200
Sugar-free foods, 201
Supergirl Hamstring Curl (Glute
  Raise / Overhead Shoulder Press /
  Hamstring Curl / Overhead
  Triceps Extension), 129
Superman, 111

Advanced, 140
  Beginning, 77
Super Speed Skate, 155
Super Squat (Squat / Overhead
  Shoulder Press / Close Squat /
  90-Degree Chest Fly), 132
Support-group meetings, 257
Support system, 17
Swayback posture, 9
Sweets, 199–200. See also Dessert recipes

Tai chi, 50
Target heart rate, 57
Tendonitis, 176–177
Torso Hang, 162
Total-Body Circuit Workouts, 52
Tough-Girl Push-up, 110
Towels, 4
Trans fats, 194–195, 199
Travel, workout program during, 22
Triceps Extension, 96
  Overhead, 65, 129
Triceps Kickback, 85, 137
Triceps Kickback / Bent-Over Row, 109
Triceps Stretch, 164
Trouble Spots Workout, 52
Tuck Jack, 154

Undereating, 211
Unsaturated fats, 194
Upright Row, 66, 135
Uptown Arms (Overhead Front Raise /
  Overhead Triceps Extension), 96

Vegetarian proteins, 192
Vitamins, 188

Waist-to-hip ratio, 12
Warm-ups, 179
Water, 197–199
Water bottle, 3
Weekly goals, 25
Weighing, 40–42
Weight, obsession with, iv
Weight loss
  as a goal 25, 26
  mental side of, 15–20
Weight-loss pills, 187–188
Weight training, 48
Windmill Plank (Plank / Side Plank), 147
Wine, 197
Workout boredom, 251–252
Workout form, proper, 181
Workout journals, 29–31, 37
Workout moves
  Level I, 59–93
  Level II, 94–125
  Level III, 126–158
Workout notes, 30
Workout plans, 45
Workout program, 45–51
  commitment to, 21–22
  levels of, 52–54
  making time for, 22
  while traveling, 22
Workout time, increasing, 181

Yoga, 50